A
PAIN
IN THE NECK

By
Arthur Winter, M.D., F.I.C.S
Director, New Jersey Neurological Institute
&

Ruth Winter, M.S.

A Pain In The Neck
The Latest Information on Causes, Therapies, Prevention

ASJA Press
an imprint of iUniverse, Inc.

iUniverse books may be ordered through booksellers or by contacting:

iUniverse
2021 Pine Lake Road, Suite 100
Lincoln, NE 68512
www.iuniverse.com
1-800-Authors (1-800-288-4677)

Originally published by WiseGuide Publishing

ISBN: 0-595-34920-X

Printed in the United States of America

Other Books
By The Authors

Vitamin E: *Your Protection Against Exercise Fatigue, Weakened Immunity, Heart Disease, Cancer, Aging, Diabetic Damage, Environmental Toxins.* Crown, January 1998.

Brain Workout: *Easy Ways to Power Up Your Memory, Sensory Perceptions & Intelligence.* Co-authored with Arthur Winter, M.D., St. Martin's Press, 1997.

Anti-Aging Hormones: *Benefits & Dangers of The Chemicals That Can Help You Beat The Clock: Melatonin, Human Growth Hormone, DHEA, Estrogen, Testosterone, Leptin, Thymosin, Thyroid, and Growth Factors.* Crown, July 1997.

Super Soy: *The Miracle Bean.* Crown, 1996 (Doubleday Book Club)

A Consumer's Guide To Medicines In Food: *Nutraceuticals That Help Prevent and Treat Emotional and Physical Ills.* Crown, May 1995 (Book-of-the-Month Club).

A Consumer's Dictionary of Food Additives. Crown, 1974. Revised 1976. Revised 1984. Revised 1989. Revised October 1994.

A Consumer's Dictionary of Cosmetic Ingredients. Crown, 1974. Revised 1976. Revised 1984. Revised 1989. Revised 1994.

A Consumer's Dictionary of Household, Yard and Office Chemicals. Crown Publishers, July 1992 (Literary Guild Book Club).

A Consumer's Guide To Free Medical Information By Phone and By Mail. Prentice Hall. February 1993 co-author Arthur Winter, M.D.

A Consumer's Dictionary of Prescription, Non-Prescription, Homeopathic, & Herbal Medicines. Crown Publishers, January 1994, 1996.

Poisons In Your Food. Revised 1991 (Beware of The Foods You Eat Revised and updated edition of Poisons In Your Food, 1969) Poisons In Your Food, Crown, 1971, NAL, 1971.

This book describes current information about neck problems, diagnosis and therapy but it is not a substitute for your doctor.

For further information about health, nutrition, cosmetics, brain and memory function, please visit our website at:

www.BrainBody.com

CONTENTS

INTRODUCTION

Your neck is a very sensitive barometer of your physical and emotional well being since it provides a vital link between your brain and the rest of your body. It is exquisitely vulnerable to stresses and strains both within you and in the environment around you.

As a neurosurgeon, I have found that the more you understand, the more effectively you can deal with problems that arise. Your input is vital to the diagnosis because the neck can sometimes be a very subtle offender. Its dysfunction can cause such varied symptoms as dizziness, headaches, blurred vision, or numbness in a limb.

This text is an explanation of the causes and results of problems that relate to your neck. They are described in accurate but understandable language. Many preventive and corrective means are given, including an outline of exercises that may be beneficial in maintaining optimal strength and normal conditions of your neck. The usual medical and surgical procedures are explained, as well as their indications and results.

Almost everyone at one time or another suffers a "pain in the neck." Quite often, only simple measures are required to prevent or to treat the condition. This book explains the common causes, therapies, and methods of avoiding neck problems. However, you must be aware that this is only a guide. When any of the symptoms described in the book are severe, prolonged, or resistant to treatment, see your own physician!

Chapter 1

NO WONDER YOUR NECK HURTS

A forty-two-year-old newspaper editor raced against time to check the proofs of a series of articles exposing a political payoff situation in his city. He had been sitting at his desk without a break for five hours, his head bent over his work. A pencil slipped to the floor and he bent to pick it up. Suddenly, the room began to spin. Ike felt sick to his stomach and a pain shot from his shoulder down to the wrist of his left arm.

"It must be a heart attack or a stroke," he thought with utter dismay. But it wasn't. The editor was suffering from a common occupational hazard, neck strain. Computer users, hair stylists, bookkeepers, dentists, surgeons, cooks and, in fact, all people who must keep their heads in one position for long periods of time are particularly prone to this malady.

You have at present or probably have had a pain in the neck. Most of us have had the experience of awakening with a painful stiff neck or being struck by a sudden pain when turning our heads. Have you ever had difficulty raising your hand to comb your hair because of neck discomfort? Few of us escape such aches and for a very basic reason, the way we are made.

Remember the man with a stick on his forehead in the circus who balanced a goldfish bowl on the other end of the stick? Well, his job was not much different from that of your neck. It balances the weight of your head, which is about seven pounds, on seven triangular bones called vertebrae. The first vertebra, the one at the top, is called the *atlas* after the Greek god in mythology who supported the world on the back of his neck and shoulders. The second vertebra is called the *axis* because it has a toothlike projection upon which the *atlas* and your

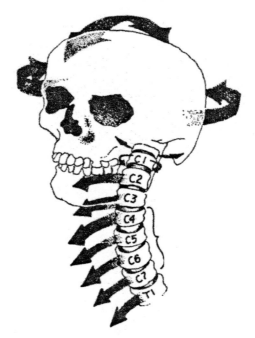

Relationship of head and neck movements

head rotate.

The devastating injury suffered by Christopher Reeve, the actor who played Superman, involved the *atlas* and the *axis*. He was thrown from his horse and landed on his head damaging these top two vertebrae. Without immediate and expert care he would not have survived the injuries since he was then unable to breathe on his own.

Under ordinary circumstances, the *atlas* and the *axis* are somewhat protected. They are nestled under your skull and thus are less vulnerable to stress than the remaining five vertebrae of your neck. These five bones lie in the center of your neck, which must, like the circus juggler, balance your heavy head on the twelve relatively immobile chest vertebrae attached to your ribs.

Your head and neck move almost continuously during your waking hours. Your neck must have a wide range of motions in all directions because of your head's special sense organs of sight and hearing. You shake and rotate your head on your neck to see, hear, nod "yes," shake "no," avoid a glance, concentrate on a sight, or do any of the myriad of gestures for which you use the anatomy above your shoulders.

Moving your head for you are thirty-two highly complex muscles and numerous elastic ligaments. In addition to rotating your head, neck muscles also control your chewing, swallowing, and facial expression.

Your muscles, of course, work by moving the column of your neck bones. The movement below the number one *atlas* and the number two *axis* is that of gliding. Your neck bones actually function in pairs. The third glides upon the fourth and the fourth upon the fifth, and so on. They work together on

3

sort of roller-bearing joints while remaining separated by a tough-on-the-outside, soft-on the-inside cushion called a *disc*. The front part of the pair of bones where the disc is located is primarily weight bearing and shock absorbing.

Meanwhile, in the middle through the narrow, vulnerable tunnel formed by the arches of your seven neck bones (vertebrae), runs your spinal cord, the vital communication line between your brain above and the rest of your body below. To the left and right of this main tunnel are two smaller tunnels in which your big vertebral arteries wend their way, carrying blood up from your heart to nourish parts of your spinal cord and brain. Your jugular vein is also at home in the neck and so are your carotid arteries, which feed your brain, face, and eyes. Insults to any of these vital blood carriers may cause you to have a potpourri of symptoms ranging from dizziness, palpitation, and ringing in the ears to fainting, mental difficulties, blind-

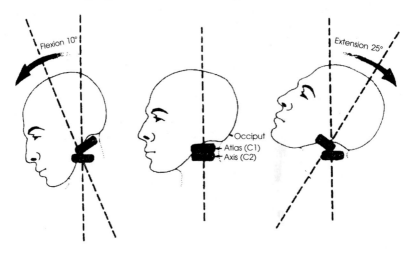

Modification of cervical vertebrae (neck bones)
with different head positions.

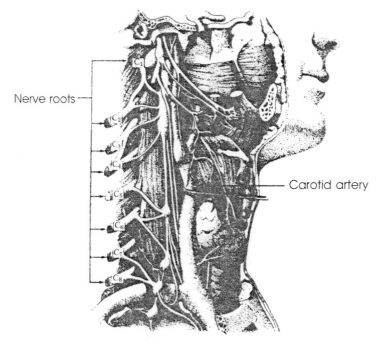

Nerve roots

Carotid artery

Nerves and arteries of the neck.

ness, paralysis of the limbs, and even death. The clogging by fat deposits of a neck artery, which feeds the brain, is a common cause of stroke, which in turn may lead to speech problems, and degrees of paralysis.

As if the afore mentioned vital structures were not enough responsibility for your fragile neck, it also contains your pharynx (throat), larynx (voice box), thyroid gland (regulator of body chemistry), trachea (windpipe), epiglottis (windpipe safety valve), esophagus (food pipe), tonsils and your other lymph glands, and the base of your tongue. Disease or malfunctioning of any of these structures may cause a pain in your neck.

Controlling all these muscles and many other vital functions in your body are the nerves in your neck. These nerves derive from the spinal cord that is monitored and controlled by your brain.

Your vagus nerve, which descends into your neck through an opening in your skull, has fibers, which reach and affect your heart, lungs, larynx, stomach, intestines, liver, pancreas, spleen, and kidneys. Your phrenic nerve, which emanates from

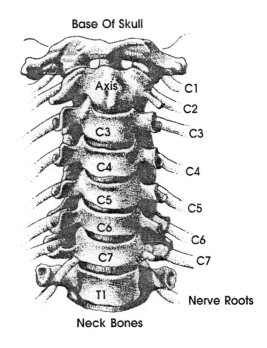

Vertebrae (neck bones) and nerve roots.

the spinal cord in your neck, controls your diaphragm, the main muscle of breathing.

Ironically, most of the time when something is wrong with your neck, the pain is felt in another part of your body. Headache, shoulder pain, and dizziness are probably the most common symptoms, but any mechanical ailment or pain may lead back to that space between your head and shoulders.

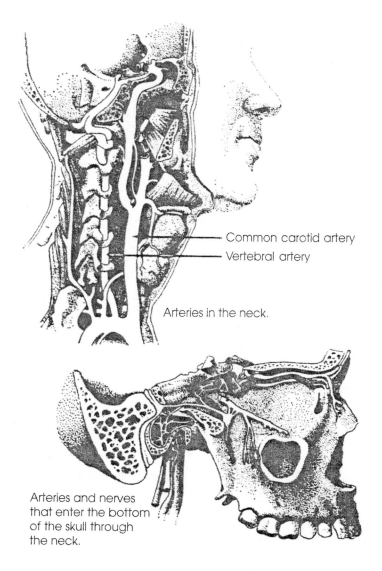

Common carotid artery
Vertebral artery

Arteries in the neck.

Arteries and nerves
that enter the bottom
of the skull through
the neck.

Because your neck has such influence in remote places in
your body, it is sometimes difficult to make a diagnosis; how-

ever, much work in tracing the route of neck-caused pain has been done in recent years, and the road map can easily be read by physicians once the proper clues have been given.

Pain that starts in the superficial structures of the neck, the skin or muscle, is most often associated with local soreness directly at the site. Pain, which emanates from the deeper structures, the bone, nerves, or deep-lying blood vessels, is usually felt over a wider area, often without a specific identifiable point of pain.

By listening to the history of your pain and just where you are currently feeling the distress, a physician has a good clue about the cause of your trouble, even if that cause is far removed from the actual trouble spot. For instance, a pain in the sixth neck bone (cervical vertebra, C6) can cause pain in your shoulder, arm, or hand.

Your nerves enter and leave your spinal cord via passages in your neck bones. Their duty is to receive messages and to send them to your brain. At the same time, they receive messages from your brain and relay orders to control your neck, shoulder, arm, and hand movements. If your neck nerves are not receiving the messages properly, you may feel numbness, pain, or loss of temperature sensation in your neck, shoulder and arm, or hand. If the neck nerves are not sending messages correctly. You may have partial or total paralysis of any of these structures.

The nerves of your neck bones are connected to your skin in sort of a road-map fashion. The travel routes by which they receive information are laid out in a pattern called *dermatomes*. The stimuli's messages are picked up by the nerve endings in your skin and sent by nerve "wire" to the neck nerves, which

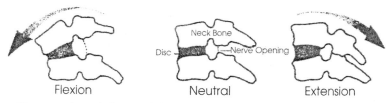

Flexion | Neutral | Extension

Compression of disc and shape related to cervical bones (neck) during movement.

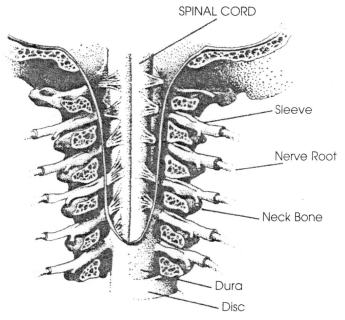

Cutaway revealing nerve and bone structures.

then relay the messages to your spinal cord and finally your brain for interpretation and reaction. The neck nerves and skin sites that act as "radio receivers" for them are shown in the following chart.

Neck Nerves And Skin Sites

Nerve Root	Skin Site
C1	Back of head
C2	Back of the head and neck
C3	Upper part of the neck
C4	Upper shoulder and collar bone
C5	Middle part of shoulder
C6	Arm and hand to thumb and index finger
C7	Forearm and third finger
C8*	Back of forearm and third and fourth fingers
T1†	Hand and fifth finger

* Although there are only seven neck bones there are eight neck nerve roots.

† T1 is the first nerve from the thorax but its function overlaps with the neck nerves because it affects the hand and finger.

The neck nerves with the specific movements they control are shown in the chart on page 12.

Pain on movement in every direction suggests trouble within the joints or parts directly connected with it. Ability to move freely in most directions, but not all, gives a clue that the lesion is in a specific group of structures outside the joint proper, such as the skin or muscle.

Pain when resistance is deliberately applied to the movement, such as trying to move your arm while someone is holding it, leads to the conclusion that the problem is in the muscle or tendon. The tendon is the tough, strong band that transmits the power of the muscle to the bone.

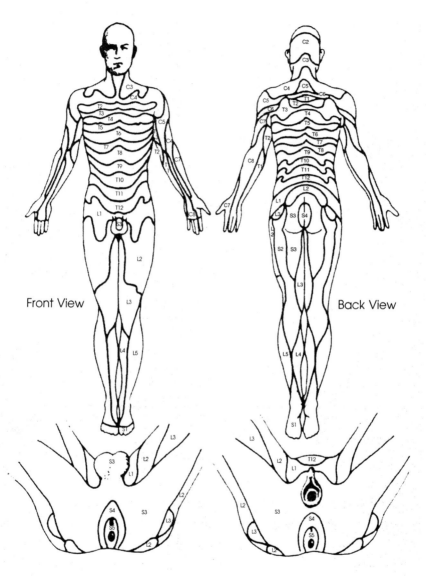

Front View

Back View

Body Dermatomes and relationship to nerves.

11

Neck Nerves And Movement

Nerve	Joint	Movement
C3, C4	shoulder	Shrugging
C5, C6	shoulder	moving arm away
		lateral rotation
	elbow	flexion
		straightening arm out
		extension
C6, C7, C8	shoulder	moving arm toward self
		medial rotation
		flexion
		extension
C7, C8	wrist	flexion
	thumb and fingers	extension
	joints of fingers	flexion
		extension
C7, C8, T1	thumb	moving toward body
		flexion
C8, T1	thumb	flexion
		moving toward body
		opposition
	fingers	flexion
		moving toward and
		away from body

The causes of neck, arm, shoulder, and hand pain emanating from the neck may be due to injury, disease or just to the vulnerability of our necks as we go about our days and sleep in our beds at night. Diagnosis of the source of such pain is made by a careful history, X-rays, electrical tests, imaging tests, and physical examination.

While almost everyone suffers from neck-related pain sometime or other, and such pain can range from mild to excruciating, fortunately there is much that can be done by physicians and a considerable amount that can be done by you to prevent these problems.

CHAPTER 2

WHEN WEAR AND TEAR GIVE YOU A PAIN IN THE NECK

We start out with a neck that is engineered to take stress and strain. First of all, the neck, like the back, has a forward curve. If these curves were not present and we were ramrod straight from head to toe, every step we took would telegraph a jolt to our brains. Running and jumping would literally beat our brains out.

The very objects that fashion these curves, the intervertebral discs, are designed to help absorb the jolts and to keep us moving easily. The discs are set between the neck and backbones. Each disc is a flattened, cushion-like sac with an outer wall of tough, fibrous connective tissue. The contents of the sac, the *nucleus pulposus*, looks almost exactly like crabmeat when healthy and like gelatin dessert when not. Wider in the front than in the back, the discs when lined up give our neck and low back those forward

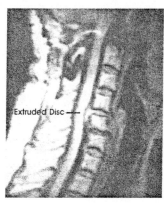

MRI of an extruded disc

13

curves.

Discs are compressible and permit us to rotate and tilt our heads as well as to nod them forward and bend them back. But when a disc slips out from between two bones, we have a ruptured disc.

Aging and repeated mechanical injury in the form of constant motion and weight bearing cause degeneration of the discs, Joint of Luschka, and bones (vertebrae) in the neck. They lose their normal firm elasticity and tend to become soft, friable, and granular. In fact, disc disease is estimated to be the major cause of neurological problems emanating from the neck.

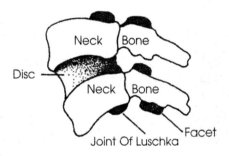

Almost all neck X-rays of people over thirty-five show a narrowed interspace between the neck bones demonstrating loss of disc substance. This is most evident at C5 and C6 and next at C6 and C7, and then at C4 and C5, the areas of the neck that are involved in most motion and therefore in the most abuse.

What happens when a disc ruptures or protrudes from its nesting place between the neck bones?

The disc may interfere with the opening through which the neck nerves pass. The nerve root and its accompanying tissues fill half of the opening and the space remaining is very vulnerable to compression.

The gluey jelly of the ruptured disc does not disintegrate easily and absent itself from causing trouble. The pressure between the bones, once borne by the disc, remains, maintained by the weight of the body and the pulling of the spinal muscles. The pressure closes the space between the bones and does not allow the disc to return to its former resting place without a struggle.

If the disc pushes out and presses on the nerve root, the nerve hurts. Inflammation occurs and causes swelling and interference with the blood supply within the nerve roots. Sometimes the mechanical presence of the extruded disc material is not as harmful as the inflammation that it causes. The inflammation may last a long time, and a scar may be produced within the nerve root or between the root and its surrounding tissue and produce chronic neck pain.

Most patients who have a neck-disc problem give a history of having had an injury to the neck in a car or while participating in a sport. But not always. One doctor reported seeing many people who led sedentary lives and had severe neck-disc problems, while a fifty-year-old professional stock car driver with a history of more than twenty head and neck injuries showed normal disc spaces when X rayed.

An acute problem where the disc suddenly pops out during a trauma to the head or neck or during strenuous exercise is not hard to diagnose. The victim is most likely between thirty and fifty years old. He complains of severe pain that developed out of the blue at the base of the neck and radiated down to the arm, shoulder, and forearm. The more common and more subtle disc problems, which tend to occur in the older age group, are more difficult to pinpoint because the symptoms may be vague and diverse.

The victim usually complains of a stiff neck for some years. At first the symptoms are attributed to a cool draft or to charley horse. As time goes by, the pain increases. Sneezing, changing positions, or coughing may cause intense discomfort. The pain radiates from the shoulder down to the fingers, following the road map of nerves, which was mentioned previously.

Pain when moving the neck forward or when turning the head to one side tells a tale of a disc. When touched lightly with a piece of cotton on the arm or shoulder, such persons frequently show a loss of sensitivity giving a further clue to blockage of nerve transmission in the neck.

With the disc problem developed over the years, only one disc may have moved or ruptured, but frequently many discs are involved, giving the person's neck the look of a washboard on an X-ray picture. All the discs protrude to some degree.

About eighty percent of all patients with cervical disc disease can be managed adequately by conservative therapy, bed rest, aspirin, and muscle relaxants prescribed by a physician. If this still does not help, surgery may be necessary to remove the disc and to relieve the pressure on the nerve.

When Arthritis Gets You In The Neck

Just as the discs in the neck are affected by wear and tear as the years go by, so are the bones. Middle-aged and elderly people complain of a snapping and grating of the neck. That is usually due to osteoarthritis changes which can be seen easily on X rays in most people over forty. This most common form of joint disorders first appears without symptoms in the twenties and thirties and becomes universal by age 70 years. Almost all of us by age 40 have some pathologic changes in weight-bearing joints, including those of the neck.

Osteoarthritis is a degenerative condition caused by repeated injury to the joints. It is so common and so ancient that even those long-necked dinosaurs show it in their bones.

The cartilage and other tissues that make the joints move properly break down. The damage from osteoarthritis is confined to the joint and surrounding tissues. There is little or no inflammation but there is pain and a limiting of normal movement.

The ends of the bones are designed to fit snugly together. The end of each bone is covered with a layer of smooth, rubberlike gristle, the cartilage. The joint cartilage acts as an elastic cushion and with proper lubrication permits our bones to move in easy harmony.

In all joints, the ends of the bones are attached by sheets and strands of tough fibers called ligaments. The ligaments of an osteoarthritis joint are more susceptible to sprain than the ligaments of a normal joint. Each joint is completely enclosed in a capsule of similar tissue. The capsule is lined by a membrane that secretes a lubricating fluid into the space between the bones. This lubricant is called *synovial fluid*.

The first noticeable change as osteoarthritis arrives is a softening, pitting, and fraying of the smooth cartilage surface. It loses its elasticity and becomes more vulnerable to further damage and stress and strain. As the disease progresses, whole sections of cartilage may be worn away completely, leaving only smooth bone ends exposed to each other. When the gliding surfaces of cartilage are gone, it may become painful to move the joint, and the joint may begin to lose its normal shape. The underlying bone ends become thickened and bony spurs may form where the ligaments and capsules are attached. Cysts, fluid-filled bubbles, may form near the joint, and fragments of bone or cartilage can become loose within the joint.

In very severe osteoarthritis, the normal shape and mechanical structure of the joint may be destroyed. The neck may literally become stiff.

Primary arthritis starts by itself. No one knows why. Secondary arthritis occurs after an injury. Football players get it in the knees, ballet dancers in the ankles, and we all get it, to some degree, in the neck.

Ballet dancers and football players get it because they use those joints so much. But not all football players or ballet dancers get osteoarthritis. Most of us do get osteoarthritis, but some of us don't. Why?

No one knows for sure why some people with the same occupation or same history of injury get osteoarthritis while others do not. One theory is that some people just have better cartilage than others do. Another theory is that there is some as yet undetected chemical abnormality that causes the damage. The only two mammals that don't appear to suffer from it are bats and sloths that spend much of their lives hanging upside down.

The pain of osteoarthritis is caused by irritation and pressure on nerve endings, muscle tension and muscle fatigue.

In some cases, called *spondylosis*, the disc spaces are narrowed and the disc material bulges outward in all directions like a fat man sitting on a cushion. Above and below the discs new bone forms called *osteophytes*. Along with the bulging discs, the bone spurs may compress the spinal canal and nerves. Usually gradual in onset, spondylosis, like osteoarthritis, is slow and progressive. There is less flexibility in the neck. Eventually it becomes difficult to fully rotate the head, and the muscles are tender.

If you have moderate arthritis of your neck, chances are a physician in his or her office or clinic can treat you. Muscle relaxants, heat, gentle massage, home cervical traction, and injections of anesthetic are used. If the pain is severe and/or there is growing weakness and perhaps paralysis, you should be seen by a physician to determine the cause and possible urgent need for surgery.

The object of medical treatment is to control pain and to protect the joints from further stresses and strains. Splints, braces, and exercises may be employed. All agree, the sooner rehabilitative methods are employed the more of your neck's flexibility and your motor strength can be preserved. There also will be less damage to your arms and shoulders.

CHAPTER 3

BREAK NECK SPORTS

From the playing fields of football to the diving boards of swimming pools, the neck is always in danger. Between 10,000 and 20,000 persons sustain a spinal cord injury in the United States each year. Approximately one-half of these injuries result in quadriplegia (loss of movement in arms and legs) and one-half sustain paraplegia (loss of movement in legs.) According to the American Association of Neurosurgeons and the Congress of Neurosurgeons, the leading causes include:

> ➢ Motor vehicle crashes account for up to 60 percent of spinal cord injuries.
> ➢ Falls.
> ➢ Acts of violence.
> ➢ Sports.
> ➢ Diving accounts for 66 percent of sports injuries.
> ➢ Alcohol is a contributing factor in about 40 percent of injuries.
> ➢ Children 15 years and under sustain up to 14 percent of spinal cord injuries; one-third of which occur when youngsters are playing or are engaged in sports.

The neck is one of the most vulnerable areas of an athlete's body. The injury to the neck may be mild and temporary, or it may be incapacitating or even fatal. One of the problems with a severely injured neck, including a broken one, is that symptoms may appear immediately or not until hours later. Therefore, an immediate diagnosis should be made. Efforts in rescue should be to prevent further damage to the spinal cord or nerves.

Take the classic case of a Princeton football player. During a game in Palmer Stadium against Dartmouth, a captain of the Tigers brushed off two blockers and made a head-on tackle of a halfback.

Although the captain didn't know it at the time, he had received an "explosive fracture" of the atlas. In other words, he had shattered the first neck bone on which the head rests. He stayed in for two more plays and then took himself out of the game.

The full extent of his injury became known the next day when X-rays showed the break. Emergency surgery was performed and metal pincers were placed in his skull above the ears like tongs holding a piece of ice. Weights were attached to the pincers to keep his head straight until his neck had a chance to mend.

The halo technique is used in most cases of broken necks for stabilization and to permit ambulation. Before its development, nearly all victims died because of dislocation of vertebrae with pressure and damage to the spinal cord.

The Princeton captain stayed in the hospital for almost a year before he was released in a body cast. The cast was later replaced by a neck brace to support his head. Three years after the accident, he was well enough to attend medical school.

He was very, very lucky. A break in the neck that injures or severs the spinal cord may paralyze all or some of the body's functions, including breathing. Death can be quick or slow, depending on the part of the spinal cord injured. Once the cord is cut, as of this writing, there is no hope for recovery of the functions lost. But with proper care, an injured cord may recover all or some of its former capabilities.

Foot ball players' necks are frequently traumatized. In fact, it is estimated that five percent of players in the U.S. sustain neck injuries each year. In one year alone, nineteen football fatalities were directly related to head and neck injuries.

It has been shown that the force against the football helmet when a player crashed into an opponent is five thousand times the force of gravity, and it is the neck which takes the brunt of that force.

Spearing techniques once often used in football have been ruled out although such injuries may occur in unsupervised games. The players deliberately use their heads as battering rams. The maneuver is dangerous both for the player and for the person he hits.

Another very common injury in football is due to a player being hit in such a way that his head is forced sideways. It is called a *lateral flexion injury*. There is immediate pain from the base of the neck to the hand, with a tingling sensation in the arm and perhaps an inability to move it. In a short time these sensations disappear leaving in their wake a dull ache in the neck and shoulder.

Many players shrug off the pain, pull themselves together,

and re-enter the game. By the time the real extent of the injury is detected, damage may be considerable and the victim is painfully aware that the symptoms were not mild and temporary.

The players most likely to suffer this type of injury are blocking backs or interior linemen with average builds and neck flexibility. The players with short, thick muscular necks are not often victims. Therefore, athletes with long, thin necks should not play football.

The result of the lateral flexion injury is commonly called a *pinched nerve*, but this is not quite accurate. The problem is actually the result of an over-stretching of the neck nerves and ligaments when the shoulder is forced downward as the head is driven to the opposite side, usually after receiving a body block. The severity depends upon the degree of stretching of the nerves and ligaments.

The pain in the neck and shoulder may be severe, and neurological changes in the arm are common. The muscle reflexes may diminish and numb spots may develop and last for several months. Occasionally muscle weakness of the shoulder and hand persist for more than a year. Associated with these findings may be a limitation of the neck movement toward the affected side due to swelling, scarring and compression of the nerve root.

To protect against neck injuries in football, doctors recommend that youngsters with long, thin necks choose another sport. Those with short, muscular necks are best suited for the game, but even they should strengthen their neck muscles against assault with exercise (see Chapter 13).

Diving into Disaster

Another sport, which is dangerous to the neck, is diving. Each year, about 1000 diving-related injuries occur. This accounts for 10 percent of spinal cord injuries and 60 percent of all recreational injuries. Ninety-five percent of all diving injuries in pools occur in five feet of water or less. Minor injuries are less frequent than in football, but when accidents do occur, the consequences are usually more serious and may include paralysis and death.

The American Association of Neurological Surgeons and the Congress of Neurological Surgeons have established a program called THINK FIRST that provides the following advice to protect yourself and your loved ones against diving injuries:

- ➢ Check the depth of the water and learn how deep it is as well as where the rocks, sandbars, or other objects may be located.
- ➢ Don't drink and dive. Many diving injuries are related to drinking.
- ➢ When body surfing, choose the beach carefully and know the wave patterns. When coming to shore, avoid surfing headfirst and roll horizontal to the waves.

Diving injuries always happen because the swimmer has dived into shallow water or struck his head against an object. The skull receives the brunt of the impact, but the neck is violently flexed and dislocated or fractured and the swimmer may drown.

When a person hurts himself diving, always assume that the neck is broken. It is better to be safe than sorry. A broken neck is a dire emergency, one in which well-meaning first-aiders can do a great deal of harm. More than five hundred persons a year are rendered totally paralyzed from the neck down because they were given improper first aid in a diving accident.

Your first instinct is to pull a victim from the water to prevent drowning. Many people do it by pulling the person's hair. Don't do it!

Do the following:

1) Jump into the water and support the victim's body in the water in as straight a line as possible.
2) Wait until a hard surface has been obtained, such as a surfboard, door, or stretcher. The support must be even and not susceptible to bending or breaking - styrofoam paddle boards or inflated mattresses should not be used.
3) Tie the person to the board before bringing him out of the water. A large beach towel, several bound together bathrobe ties, or rope may be used. If only one tie is available, use it to encircle the chest area.

Because neck injuries in diving accidents are common, life guards and persons with backyard pools should have as standard equipment a spine (hard) board as well as life preservers. Remember, a person involved in a diving accident should be "splinted where he floats" before attempting to remove him from the water.

Riding accidents

Falls off horses are common, in fact, even the best horsemen tumble off once in a while. But if the rider pitches onto his head, an injury to the neck may occur. Christopher Reeve, the 6"4' actor and expert horseman, still is not sure what happened that day in Culpeper, Virginia, in 1995, when his horse halted suddenly before an easy, three-foot jump. Reeve said his hands became entangled in the bridle, so that he could not break his fall. He landed on his head, the force of his 200-pound body fracturing his first and second cervical vertebrae. He was paralyzed and unable to breathe on his own. He was wearing a helmet. The skulls of most riders today are protected by helmets so the brain escapes serious injury, but the rider may still injure his or her neck as in the Reeve case. Fortunately, most riding accidents are not that devastating.

Race Car Driving

There are many devastating accidents with racecar drivers. In 1997, a device developed by a Michigan University engineer known as HANS (head and neck support) was worn in the Indianapolis 500 Memorial Day Race. It is a combination helmet and yoke that supports a driver's head, helps reduce neck fatigue and avoid the accompanying injuries common among drivers. More than 250 race drivers are now wearing them and perhaps similar devices may be used in other sports and even someday by the rest of us under certain circumstances.

Judo and karate

The increasing interest in these self-defense sports is causing a growing number of neck injuries.

Judo. The somersaults and falls cause an over-extension of the neck, particularly when unexpected. Total body weight on the head and neck during a fall can result in a simple neck sprain or a broken neck and spinal cord injury.

Karate. Direct blows to any part of the neck can cause local trauma, hemorrhage, and sudden death. This is due to the sharp edge of the hand against the soft structures of the neck. The force of the blow may be transmitted to the spinal cord and other vital structures.

Cycling and gymnastics

Cycling, particularly motorcycling, and gymnastics also put the vulnerable neck in danger. Cycling, for the same, reason as horseback riding - the victim may pitch over onto his or her skull, jarring the neck.

Gymnastics, because of all the peculiar twists, turns and aerial acrobatics taken during execution of the events. A wrong twist, turn or fall may lead to the neck being injured or even broken. Careful supervision and training is imperative to protect against serious injury in this sport.

Hunting

Another sport in which a life-threatening injury to the neck may occur is hunting. A bullet may accidentally be shot through the neck, although this type of injury most often occurs during war or the commission of a crime. It is due to wars, those of the Korean and Vietnam vintage, that immediate care of such wounds has improved dramatically. In previous times, people with a bullet or knife wound in the neck usually died from a blocked airway or from uncontrolled bleeding.

Remember, any wound of the neck is serious. Even if the skin wound at the point of entrance appears innocuous to you, a minor cut may hide a lethal injury. Medical attention should be sought at once. In the meantime, pressure should be applied to the wound to stop hemorrhaging, and mouth-to-mouth resuscitation should be given if breathing stops.

How Do You Know It's Serious?

When it is understood that the neck can easily be injured during sports and that proper first aid treatment is essential, a lot of suffering might be avoided and many lives could be saved each year.

As mentioned before, a broken neck or back is a dire emergency. How do you know there is a break? You don't for sure, but ask the victim to move his fingers and toes. If he can't, assume there is cord injury, be careful! If he has a tingling sensation or numbness in his extremities or pain when he tries to move them, a break in the neck or backbones may have occurred.

Loosen the clothing around the victim's neck and waist. Cover him to prevent shock. Do not move the *victim* for any reason. Remember that the spinal cord extends through the neck and backbones. Any movement or pressure may cause permanent paralysis or death. Expert manipulation and transportation is usually relegated to the emergency crew of an ambulance. Always call 911 for the proper instructions before moving a victim unless even more danger is imminent such as speeding cars, flooding, or blowing objects. If for some absolute necessity the victim must be moved without professional assistance, it must be done with the utmost care. A hard, straight surface must be used, such as a board or door, just as in a diving accident.

Do not take a chance with anything that may sag or collapse. Place the board next to the person. Every part of the body should be supported. It is vital the body be kept in a straight line without bending, as pointed out above. The board should be slipped under the victim, and the person should then be tied or held on the board so there is a minimum of movement and transferred in a flat position, not seated.

CHAPTER 4

WHIPLASH
THE DANGEROUS JERK

Mention the word *whiplash* and most adults will picture a passenger in an automobile that is hit from behind by another car while his own vehicle is at a standstill. The passenger's head and neck are thrown forward or backward, with recoil in the opposite direction.

Actually, any movement, which produces an over-extension or a deep recoil of the neck, may cause a whiplash. Dr. John Caffey of the University of Pittsburgh, the pediatric radiologist who first made the nation aware of the battered-child syndrome, reported at .an American Medical Association meeting that the harried mother who shakes her infant to make it stop crying, or to correct its behavior may be risking brain damage and even mental retardation in her child because she, or often "her boyfriend", is giving the baby a whiplash.

Dr. Caffey said the danger period for most infants is the first year of life, particularly the first six months when the brain is still soft and immature before the skull has solidified. At this age, also, the baby's head is relatively heavy and his neck muscles weak, so that shaking produces the whiplash action that bumps the brain against the inside of the skull. Pinpoint hemorrhages and damage to the blood vessels may result in serious or fatal injury to the infant.

The syndrome has now become recognized so often, it is has its own name, "Shaken Baby Syndrome."

Our skulls become thicker and our necks a little stronger as we mature, but we are all vulnerable to the effects of whiplash suffered by the shaken babies. Even tripping and catching ourselves with an outstretched hand, or just landing suddenly on the buttocks, can jolt the neck. Furthermore, snapping of the head from side to side can cause a whiplash just as the front-to-back recoiling can.

The whole subject of whiplash injury is fraught with controversy, particularly as it applies to automobile accidents. Its consequences range from frequent permanent damage to the neck, caused by even slight whiplash, to a pain in the pocketbook which is cured only by a successful court suit.

Some physicians and lawyers refuse to use the term *whiplash* because it has been associated with so many liability claims in court.

It has been estimated that out of every ten neck injuries doctors see, eight are the results of car accidents. In all motor-vehicle accidents, eighty-six percent of the victims reportedly have injuries to the neck.

The most common accident associated with whiplash is, of course, the rear-end collision, a phenomenon that occurs in twenty percent of all crashes. Studies at the University of Rochester demonstrated that significant neck injury can result from your car being hit by another car going only five to ten miles per hour, and that your injury will be no less severe than if the accident occurs at speeds up to thirty miles an hour.

The victim of a whiplash in an auto accident is more likely to be a woman than a man. According to a New Jersey study, the neck injury rate for women in metropolitan regions was 4.8 times, and in nonmetropolitan regions 1.7 times, that of men. Several theories have arisen to explain this. One is that women are usually riding in cars with men and are in an unprotected position in the passenger seat. Another is that woman complain more than men about such things as pain in the neck; and still another theory is that the long, slender necks of women, while nice to look at, are not as good at supporting the head as men's more muscular ones.

The symptoms of a whiplash, like other symptoms rooted in the neck, are varied and widespread.

Pain may be felt immediately after the accident occurs and be so severe that the victim thinks his neck is broken. On the other hand, pain may not be felt until hours or oven days later, becoming increasingly severe as the motion of the neck continues unrestrained.

Pain due to a whiplash may be excruciating and localized in one side of the neck. The victim tilts the head to that side. A man may he unable to use his arms to do simple things like comb his hair, fasten his collar, or shave. A woman may be unable to hook her brassiere, apply her makeup, or reach for groceries on a shelf.

The back of the neck hurts and usually so does the front in a true whiplash because the head has been snapped backward, forward, or to both sides, straining or ripping the muscles, ligaments, and tendons.

There may also he tenderness on the chest, arms, shoulders, back, and neck.

More than half the patients complain of headaches. The headache starts at the back of the neck and radiates up to the ears or to the top of the head and/or the eyes. The joints of the neck may be swollen, and there is usually some limitation of movement ranging from mild stiffness to near paralysis.

Loss of balance occurs in about fifteen of the cases and may be so severe that the victim cannot walk without aid. There is a tendency, in this instance, to fall toward the side of involvement.

Twitching of the eyelid and transitory deafness also may be present.

A strange phenomenon is that the blood pressure in the arm on the side of involvement differs ten to twenty percent from the blood pressure in the other arm. In a few cases, about five percent, the pupil is dilated on the side of involvement.

Numbness or tingling in the fingers frequently occurs.

With such telltale signs of whiplash, why is it that there is controversy in both the medical and legal fields about who has really suffered a disabling injury? The reasons:

- The symptoms may occur immediately, several hours, or several days later.
- The complaints may be hard to verify by X rays or other diagnostic tests.
- The symptoms often disappear after the case is settled in court.

A report by a Detroit surgeon, Aaron A. Farbman, published in the Journal of the American Medical Association, describes one hundred thirty-six cases of uncomplicated neck sprain. Dr. Farbman wanted to find out why some patients suffered pain only briefly and mildly, while others continued to hurt for long periods following the accident.

The Michigan doctor found that the most significant factor in the duration of pain due to simple neck sprain is emotion. The patient is much slower to overcome the pain if:

➢ He or she has a background of being nervous.
➢ Takes sedatives and tranquilizers under pressure at work or at home.
➢ Has a record of serious injuries, operations and illnesses.
➢ Has recently had a death or injury in the family.
➢ Has a history of psychiatric care.

Litigation also is an important factor in the persistence of pain, according to Dr. Farbman: "The slow process of litigation is well known. This process goes on for many months to several years. In the meantime, the patient's symptoms continue, often with increased tension, until settlement is finally reached. Litigation prolongs and aggravates the accident process syndrome."

Dr. Farbman's report coincides with those of many lawyers for insurance companies, as well as those of some physicians. They have argued that symptoms following whiplash injuries are psychologically induced by the blow, especially if the blow was unexpected, undeserved, and unseen; and also that psychological trauma is more imaginary than real.

On the other side of the coin, evidence concerning severe

34

physiologic as well as psychologic damage has been amassed.

Dr. Ayub K. Ommaya and Dr. Philip Yarnell, of the Surgical Neurology branch at the National Institute of Neurological Diseases and Strokes, subjected lightly anesthetized monkeys and chimps to whiplash by placing them in a carriage on roller skate wheels and then striking; the carriage with a piston. None of the animals received significant blows to the head. All recovered.

Yet, at autopsy, most of the animals that had been concussed had visible surface hemorrhages.

Dr. Ommaya points out that the brain is particularly vulnerable to whiplash injury because of its noncompressible soft tissue. He likens it to moving a beer glass along a counter in a straight line. The fluid will remain level. But joggle the glass and the beer will spill out.

He said that the incidence and severity of whiplash increases with the animal's brain weight, and he suspects the figures are the same for humans.

Dr. Ommaya and Dr. Yarnell investigated brain hemorrhage resulting from whiplash alone. One case was a woman who drove her car into a barrier and died eight days later. The other was a New York physician whose car was rammed by a truck, but who recovered after a blood clot on his brain had been removed during surgery. Neither had struck their heads directly.

Dr. Ommaya then tried to determine whether the neurotic symptoms displayed by certain whiplash victims, restlessness and anxiety, are related to brain damage. This was first suggested in 1961 by Dr. Fernando Torres and Dr. Sidney K. Shapiro, who studied forty-five whiplash patients and forty-five closed-head injured patients who all lost consciousness. The researchers found more abnormal electroencephalograph (EEG) readings among the whiplash patients. EEG's measure and graph the electrical waves generated by the brain.

In a book by Dr. Charles Goff and his colleagues, Dr. John O. Alden and Dr. John H. Alden, Traumatic Cervical Syndrome and Whiplash, it was pointed out that seventy-four percent of the patients who received whiplash injuries had abnormal brain-wave tracings and that such brain-wave patterns "suggest a real basis for neurosis." Furthermore, they and other experts point out that whiplash may cut off the blood supply to some areas of the brain, giving rise to emotional and other hard-to-pin-down symptoms.

Many experts also point out that older people, arthritics, and those with previous injuries or problems with the neck are more susceptible to injury from whiplash than other people, which may account for the difference in symptoms between persons involved in the same accident.

What can be done to prevent whiplash?

Be careful how you step on the brakes. Power brakes with their sudden stopping ability may jar the necks of passengers, particularly those unaware that the driver is about to step on the brake. Therefore, drivers should try to give a warning when they are about to slam on the brakes.

High-powered engines with rapid acceleration may also cause lashing of the necks of unsuspecting passengers. Therefore, jackrabbit starts should be avoided.

The safety belt is of no value in preventing the lashing effect upon the neck. The headrest may be of limited use if employed properly.

Airbags are not specifically intended to prevent neck injuries and, in fact, with children and small women, they may increase the damage to the head and neck

With the objective of preventing so many whiplash injuries, in 1969 the Federal Highway Safety Authority began requiring all new cars sold in the United States to have head restraints attached to the front seats. The headrests do prevent the backward phase of the whiplash, provided they are adjusted to be level with the base of the skull. Some short people do not use the headrests at all because they claim the devices interfere with rear vision. The headrests do not stop the forward or side lashing of the head, and a number of insurance companies have reported receiving nearly as many head-restrained as unrestrained claimants following a rear-end collision.

Forewarned is Forearmed.

Being forewarned is forearmed as far as the neck is concerned. Do the following:

- ➤ Make sure your headrest is in the proper position and you attach your seat belt every time you ride in the front seat of a car.
- ➤ Use your rear-vision mirror to check for trouble.
- ➤ If you are being tailgated, pull over and let the potential whiplasher pass.
- ➤ Try to allow room in front when stopped at a light or in traffic so that you can move forward if you see someone about to bump your car from the rear.

➢ Always drive defensively.

Summing it up, whether it is called whiplash, traumatic cervical syndrome, or any other name, the injury may be very real. The initial problem is the overstretching of the supporting ligaments of the neck, those tough fibrous bands, which tie muscle to bone. If the trauma is very severe, the crabmeat-like material between the neck bones, the intervertebral discs, may be ruptured; and if the force directed at the neck is extreme, the bones themselves may be broken.

The muscles of the neck, the nerves, and the vertebral artery may be injured causing headaches, dizzy spells, and blurred vision. The brain and spinal cord also may be injured causing a variety of neurological and psychological problems.

Whiplash can be serious. It has been found that twenty-eight percent of those with neck injuries have residual neck disabilities, and the average whiplash victim is out of work for eight weeks.

Because children's heads are larger in proportion to their bodies than adults, shaking them can cause spinal cord injury, brain hemorrhage and death.

CHAPTER 5

DIZZINESS
WHEN THINGS SPIN AROUND

It's hard to keep your balance in this world, but when there is something secretly wrong with your neck it can make you dizzy without obvious cause.

Next to pain, dizziness, or vertigo as it is medically labeled, is the most common symptom. It is that frightening sensation of spinning and falling. The walls turn and the ground suddenly seems to be dropping away.

Dizziness causes coldness, clamminess, and pallor, and thus it is often mistaken for a heart attack. Since it also evokes a frightened appearance, rigid posture, and anxiety, it is often misinterpreted as an emotional rather than a physical problem.

The nausea and vomiting that accompany vertigo are frequently believed by the victim to be the cause of the dizziness when actually they are the result of it.

How is dizziness related to the neck?

First of all, our major balance mechanism, the labyrinth system, is in the inner ear. We have an *external ear*, that flap of cartilage that adorns the side of our head and on which many women and some men place earrings. It is equipped with a funnel-shaped air passage, which is lined with hair and glands that secrete wax. The funnel guides sounds from the outside to the eardrum. Then we have a *middle ear*, an air-filled space between the drum membrane and the inner ear. The *middle ear* contains three ossicles, the smallest bones in the body, which are commonly called the *hammer, anvil,* and *stirrup*. The *hammer* is attached to the eardrum and the *stirrup* is inserted into an oval window in the inner ear. Vibration of the drum sets the bones in motion. In this way, the sound is conducted to the *inner ear.*

The drum and the bones act as a transformer which increases the energy of sound vibration at the oval window. Fortunately, the middle-ear bones are not sensitive enough to catch sounds such as those produced by the muscles of the body when they move, or by the footsteps of tiny insects.

The middle ear protects the inner ear from sounds so loud that they might be harmful. In immediate reaction to extremely loud noises, one set of muscles will tighten the eardrum so that it can't vibrate too violently while another set pulls the stirrup away from the oval window so that it won't feel the full impact of the strong sound waves.

When sound reaches the eardrum, it vibrates, the bones move, and the fluid in the inner ear is set in motion, propagating the same wave form as the original sound waves striking the eardrum. Thus, the eardrum vibration is transferred to the fluid of the coiled tubes through the middle and inner ear. The inner ear consists of:

The cochlea - a spiral shaped structure that converts sound into nerve impulses.

The semicircular canals and **vestibule** for the maintenance of body balance much like the bubble in a carpenter's level.

While the semicircular canals are not part of the hearing apparatus, they are connected with the cochlea and may be affected by diseases of the inner ear. One such common affliction is Meniere's Disease, characterized by a buzzing or roaring in the ear, deafness, and vertigo.

The vertebral arteries that carry the blood from the heart to the brain through the neck are sometimes damaged by trauma or compression due to arthritis. The result is ischemia, which is decreased blood supply and oxygen to the brain. The result may be dizziness, fainting, or stroke.

The frequency and duration of dizziness in Meniere's Disease follow no predictable pattern. An attack may last only for a few minutes or for several hours. It may or may not be accompanied by nausea and vomiting. About eighty-five percent of the Meniere's Disease victims can be treated successfully with drugs. Surgery to remove the labyrinth of one ear or ultrasonic destruction of portions of the inner ear is done as a last resort.

In addition to Meniere's Disease, there are many causes of vertigo, including:

➤ Toxic effects of drugs.
➤ Multiple sclerosis.
➤ Strokes.
➤ Tumors.
➤ Inadequate blood supply to the spinal cord and brain

can be caused by problems in the neck. In fact, more and more evidence is accumulating that the most important cause of dizziness is vascular disturbance in the neck.

When heat, massage, immobilization, or traction give immediate relief from pain and dizziness, it is probable that the symptoms are due not to Meniere's Disease but to the neck.

If the neck is stiff and the muscles are very tense, tender to pressure, and painful when moved, this is further evidence that the cause lies in the neck. And of course tension, causing tightening of the neck muscles, makes it worse.

An example of how compression of the blood vessels causes dizziness was graphically illustrated when men went to the barber chair for shaves while wearing stiff collars. Called *Barber Chair Dizziness,* the syndrome would occur when patrons bent their heads far back and turned to the side to allow the barber to shave their cheeks. This would compress the carotid artery in the neck and reduce the blood flow to the brain. In the age of sex equality, there is now a syndrome called *beauty parlor stroke.* It involves straining the neck more than 15 degrees forward or back during beauty shop shampoos, long dental appointments or painting a ceiling. Straining the neck in this manner may cause not only neck pain and dizziness, but stroke because it curtails the flow of blood flow to the brain.

Neck Injury and Dizziness

Dizziness following neck injury is a common complaint. After an injury to the neck, the muscles in the neck become tense and the neck bones are held rigid to protect against pain during movement. When this tension lasts for several months, the muscles develop permanent contractions and compression of the vulnerable large vertebral artery in the neck occurs. This, in turn, results in a lack of sufficient blood to the brain stem and inner ear, causing dizziness.

The same condition can be caused by hardening of the arteries, changes in the bone, or any mechanism that interferes with the blood supply to the brain and ears.

When there is a significant cut in the blood supply there may be hearing loss, blurred vision, nausea, vomiting, sweating, and numbness of the face. There may also be a rapid back-and-forth or up-and- down eye movement called a *nystagmus*. This eye symptom may give the clue to the correct diagnosis of a list of confusing symptoms.

Dr. Ward W. Woods and Dr. W. E. Compere, Jr., of San Diego, California, found that patients with neck injuries, predominantly whiplash, who complained of dizziness had positive electronystagmograms demonstrating true nystagmus (an electronystagmogram traces the movements of the eyes on a graph).

When the dizziness was relieved by removing the pressure from the nerves in the neck, the ENG's became normal.

Vascular Neck Pain

If the cause of dizziness is hard to diagnose, the cause of vascular neck pain is even more difficult to uncover. Patients who suffer from it complain of recurrent sore throats, swollen glands, toothaches, and a myriad of other symptoms.

Physicians treat them with antibiotics. Sometimes tonsils and teeth are extracted, or medicine is given to correct thyroid problems. Such symptoms can occur in children as young as ten and in adults older than seventy-five years. Vascular

43

neck pain is about four times as common in women as in men, and the greatest incidence occurs in the winter.

How do you know when it's vascular?

A past history of frequent migraine headaches is a good clue. So is a history of viral sore throats or ulcers in the mouth and throat. Fatigue, frustration, and tension have been found to precipitate vascular pain.

Usually the pain is deep-seated, on one side, and located in the middle of the neck radiating upward along the side of the neck (common carotid artery) to the jaw and ear.

An earache may occur on the affected side. Swallowing causes pain. The tenderness is greatest under the angle of the jaw or at the center of the neck. Often the victim erroneously thinks that it's a toothache or jaw pain. The involved carotid artery is exquisitely tender, but, strangely, there is no inflammation associated with the condition. One of the most important diagnostic clues, however, is pulsation at the point of maximum tenderness. You can feel the beating with your fingers. Compression of the superficial temporal artery in the front of the ear (next to the temple) may cause relief of pain.

Because the vascular pain is so enduring and hard to diagnose, patients may begin to believe they have cancer. Treatment consists of reassuring the victim that he or she does not have a dread disease. Mild analgesics, local heat, sedatives, antihistamines, tranquilizers, and steroids have been used to control vascular neck pain.

The blood vessels and the amount of blood they carry can cause many symptoms hard to relate to the neck. By being aware of the signs and describing them accurately to your physician, dizziness and vascular pain can be identified and treated for relief of symptoms.

CHAPTER 6

A LUMP IN THE NECK

Most neck pain is due to a mechanical injury, including those sustained in the process of aging. Such pain is annoying but not life threatening. However, sometimes infections or growths, both malignant and benign, first make their presence known by appearing as a lump or lumps in the neck.

In the lymph nodes of the neck, nature has given us an early warning system as well as a line of defense against such conditions. The lymph system is made up of a network of vessels and glandular nodes which filter, drain, and distribute a clear yellowish fluid that bathes all cells. The filter glands are called *lymph nodes*. They are small organs inserted in the lymph vessels at strategic points where they can filter out infections, catch cancer cells, and protect the remainder of the body.

Any germ can produce inflammation of one or more lymph nodes. Direct inflammation of the node itself is usually due to *streptococci* or *staphylococci* germs. However, infections of neck glands are most often the result of an infection or a problem outside the gland itself.

In children, upper respiratory infections are by far the most common cause of lumps in the neck. In both children and adults, viral infections such as the so-called kissing disease, *mononucleosis*, and *cat-scratch fever* are diagnosed by the general swelling of the neck lymph nodes they cause. German measles (Rubella) may also cause swollen neck glands, especially in children.

Then, of course, there is the *mumps*. In spite of the fact that vaccination against the infection is now possible, children and adults still get the virus that causes painful enlargement of the salivary glands. The virus lodges in a patient's saliva. After an incubation period of fourteen to twenty-four days, the mumps arrives with chills, headache, loss of appetite, and "the blahs." A low to moderate fever may last twelve to fourteen hours before involvement of the salivary gland is noted. Pain on chewing or swallowing is an early symptom. Mumps can cause, in addition to a pain in the neck, inflammation of the thyroid and thymus glands, both in the neck, and more far-flung ailments in the testes, pancreas, covering of the brain, and a number of other places.

Sick Salivary Glands

Most of the time, however, the patient recovers without ill effects from the mumps. However, another virus which also attacks the same area, the salivary glands, may also cause a pain in the neck. It is the *cytomegalovirus*. In the unborn child it is devastating, causing all sorts of gross birth defects. In the young child or adult sometimes it produces no symptoms at all or it is just a mild illness often mistaken for others. In those with compromised immune systems such as AIDS sufferers, it can cause blindness and even fatalities.

There are other problems with the salivary glands that cause a pain in the neck. If the lump in your neck enlarges when you eat and disappears when you finish, you might very well have a malfunction in the glands that help us swallow our food.

When viral or bacterial infections are the root cause of swellings in the neck, those swellings are usually tender and painful. The overlying skin may be inflamed. Swelling of the surrounding tissues may occur and it can become painful to move the neck or jaw. Usually, as soon as the underlying infection is cured, the Lymph glands return to normal. Sometimes, however, small, firm nontender knobs remain and can be felt by the bearer almost indefinitely.

In young adults, as in children, lumps in the neck usually represent a local sign of generalized disease. However, when a lump in the neck cannot be traced to a previous or current infection, particularly if the lump is not painful, then the possibility of a growth must be considered.

A number of mouth, throat, and neck cancers present themselves for the first time as a swelling in the lymph glands of the neck. Cancer cells caught by the lymph node filters most often occur in adult males who have no fever. The mass feels firm, nontender, and is usually movable, although it may later become fixed.

When an elderly person has a neck mass, chances are eight out of ten that the lump is malignant. Most such malignancies emanate from the oral cavity, throat, or lungs; cancer can be cured in its early stages and such lumps should be investigated without delay.

When the cancer cells have been spotted in a neck lymph gland of a young person, cancer of the thyroid is immediately suspected. This cancer constitutes fifty percent of all neck masses and it affects a younger age group than other neck cancers.

The thyroid gland is a butterfly-shaped organ in the front of the neck. It regulates body chemistry and affects growth and maturity. Often, the lymph gland catches the stray cancer cells when the thyroid lesion itself is extremely minute and can easily be removed. That is why it is so important to have lumps in the neck diagnosed promptly.

Viral infections can also cause the thyroid gland to swell; but sometimes the lump felt in the neck is the thyroid gland itself.

A swelling of the thyroid gland, called a *goiter*, results from iodine deficiency and used to be endemic in mountainous regions where there was insufficient iodine in the diet. A number of drugs, as well as a diet containing too much cabbage and kale, may block the manufacture of thyroid hormone and result in goiter. Goiters are particularly apt to occur at puberty and during pregnancy.

The diagnosis is not hard to make because of the location of the swelling and because uptake of a radioactive tracer gives a clear picture. Usually, treatment with iodine solves the problem. Rarely is it necessary to remove the goiter for cosmetic reasons.

There are other more serious forms of goiter. Grave's Disease, a condition characterized by growth of the thyroid and excessive secretion of the thyroid hormones causes increased body metabolism and pop eyes. The cause is unknown, but a familial tendency is often seen.

Another goiter is *toxic nodular goiter*, a condition also characterized by excessive production of thyroid hormone and one or more nodules in the thyroid. It tends to occur in the older age group. The symptoms when too much thyroid hormone is produced include nervousness, weakness, weight loss, tremor, palpitation, stare, lid lag, and bulging eyes. Unlike most neck problems, thyroid dysfunction is fairly easy to diagnose and to treat.

Not all lumps in the neck, of course, are related to benign or malignant tumors or thyroid disease. Some are harmless cysts, abnormal sacs often the result of hidden defects at birth. Usually, a lump that fluctuates in size suggests a cyst.

When a lump in the neck pulsates, it may be due to a blood vessel which has ballooned out. The balloon is a vascular malformation, a condition that is similar to a bulge in an inner tube of a tire. A physician must decide when it is all right to leave the bulge alone or when it is best to have it repaired. If surgery is necessary, the vessel is patched to keep it from rupturing, just as a tire is patched.

Severe neck pain over the back of the neck and provoked by flexion of the head may be due to a brain hemorrhage. This could be caused by a ruptured blood vessel in the brain and bleeding into the spinal canal. If these symptoms occur, seek immediate medical attention.

Other causes of lumps in the neck include blood clots, fungus infection, tuberculosis, and syphilis.

Sometimes, though very rarely, a pain in the neck may be due to a brain tumor, particularly in children. Such patients have certain symptoms that give a clue to the diagnosis. The pain does not seem to be related to movement of the head and neck. The pain is always worse on the back of the neck with radiation upward to the back of the head. It is not often accompanied by significant neck stiffness. It is usually worse upon arising in the morning, easing when the patient gets out of bed and walks around. In some patients, it becomes progressively severe with coughing or bending, which causes increased pressure in the brain, and is associated with other symptoms such as vomiting, blurred vision, or difficulty with coordination.

There may be a number of causes of neck lumps. This chapter's information cannot be all inclusive. Causes of lumps may vary according to age, gender and location. Among the questions your physician will want answered are:

> Is the lump firm?
> Is soft or pliable like a water-filled sac?
> Is it painless?
> Is your entire neck swollen?
> Where is the lump—on the front, back or side?
> Has it been increasing in size?
> What are symptoms, if any, are you experiencing?
> Do you have a rash?
> Are you having trouble breathing?

Just as it is repeated over and over again that a lump in the breast must be diagnosed and treated promptly, a lump in the neck must be investigated without delay. It may merely be a swollen lymph gland due to a minor infection, or it may not. In any event, you don't want your relatives to have a "lump in the throat" because you were too late in seeking medical advice about a lump in the neck.

CHAPTER 7

STIFF NECK
TORTICOLLIS
&
FIBROMYALGIA

Almost everyone has said at one time or another, "I have a stiff neck," and attributed it to sitting in a draft. Little is actually known about the phenomenon, but it frequently occurs in epidemics and doctors believe a virus causes it.

The typical stiff neck is sudden in onset. Moderately severe, sharp pain is felt on one or both sides of the neck upon movement. The sufferer tends to hold the head still and to turn the upper body in order to look to one side. Other than local pain, there are few other symptoms, and appetite and blood count seem normal.

Discomfort usually persists for one to three days but may continue longer. Occasionally, the patient may continue to suffer from muscle spasm.

Transmission of the ailment to volunteers by injection of whole blood from victims has been successful, but attempts to isolate the infectious agent have so far been unsuccessful.

The Torture of Torticollis

Another stiff neck, one which is more serious and equally mysterious, is called *torticollis,* from the Latin *tortus* meaning, "twisted" and "collum" meaning neck. It is the technical term for what our grandparents called *wryneck.* With torticollis, the victim's neck muscles are spasmodically contracted, particularly those muscles which are controlled by the spinal accessory nerve at the base of the skull. The head is drawn to one side and is usually rotated so that the chin points to the other side.

Children may be born with the head turned toward one shoulder due to a muscle defect or a birth injury. Torticollis, however, usually occurs between the ages of 30 to 60 years and is more common in women than in men.

Victims of trauma or disease such as encephalitis can also develop torticollis and not infrequently, emotions play a part. Take the case of a sixty-five-year-old woman who developed a *wryneck.* When doctors traced back to the cause, they found it wasn't organic. Her ninety-six-year old mother had caught her in an affair with a man and slapped her on that shoulder!

The manifestation of torticollis ranges from mild to severe. It is difficult to treat because it is not well understood. Medicines, biofeedback, and emotional support may help. Torticollis may persist for life and result in a permanently twisted neck. In about 10 to 20 percent, spontaneous recovery occurs within five years of onset, usually in the milder cases of young people. One-third of torticollis victims also have other muscular problems in the jaw or eyelids or hand.

When torticollis does occur in middle life, it may suddenly

cure itself. Treatment usually consists of muscle relaxants, psychotherapy, or, as a last resort, surgery to destroy the nerves, which cause the neck muscles to turn the head.

Actually, there is much yet to be learned about torticollis. It has been reported that wryneck may result from certain powerful psychopharmaceuticals used in psychiatric hospitals, and there are a number of researchers who believe that torticollis may result from as yet unidentified physical causes rather than psychological problems as previously believed.

Fibromyalgia and The Neck

Just as torticollis was once believed to be the result of emotional problems, so too was fibromyalgia. The term *myalgia* indicates muscle pain and *fibro* refers to the fibrous tissues, muscles, tendons, ligaments, and other "white" connective tissues. The neck is one area frequently involved.

The condition, again, occurs more in women than in men, and thus is often attributed to mental stress, poor sleep, trauma, and exposure to dampness. While women often complain of generalized muscle aches, men are reportedly more likely to have a specific area that is involved.

Proper diagnosis and supportive treatments are indicated. Sloughing it off as "just caused by tension" is not acceptable. As more is learned about the relatively newly diagnosed condition, a viral or other systemic factor may become evident. In the meantime, fibromyalgia is often treated with exercises, local injections, transcutaneous stimulation (TENS), biofeedback, anti-inflammatory medications, and steroids. Massage and low-dose anti-depressants are also prescribed. As with torticollis, the condition may spontaneously improve.

CHAPTER 8

TENSION NECKACHES AND HEADACHES

The dictionary defines headache as a pain in the head but actually, in many instances, a headache is due to a pain in the neck.

Almost all creatures on earth express emotional attitudes with their bodies. Just think of the arched back of an angry cat or the stance of a growling dog. A human is also an animal and has an analogous neck response. Muscular tension is part of our innate defense mechanism. However, sustained defense posture with excessive muscle contraction in the neck, scalp, and face may cause headache in two ways: the tight neck muscles themselves hurt; and when they go into spasm, they cut off local arteries, diminishing the blood supply to the head and neck and causing even more pain.

It is actually possible to measure the changes in the electrical activity of the neck muscles during a tension headache.

Some people, when troubled, are tense while they sleep, which explains why we may wake up in the middle of the night or in the morning with a headache.

Almost everyone has tension headaches, some more than

others, depending upon how much exposure there is to emotional stresses and the vulnerability of the neck muscles.

Muscle contraction headaches, as they are officially called, come without warning. They may last from an hour to several days and may occur once in a blue moon or several times a week.

The headaches are described as: "a tight band around my head," "throbbing," "dull," or "my head feels like it's going to burst."

Surveys have shown that the majority of tension headache victims are women who first have symptoms during the child rearing years between twenty and forty. Such women frequently have a family history of headaches. As mentioned in the whiplash chapter, women do have weaker neck muscles than men, which would make them more vulnerable to stress.

Tension headache is also the most common form of head pain in children. Family pressures, trouble at school, or problems with the neighborhood children can all cause neck-related head pain in youngsters.

Migraines And The Neck

Tension headaches may be combined with or trigger migraine headaches. Migraines affect more than fifteen million Americans. The adult migraine patient has often been described as tense, anxious, ambitious and perfectionistic.

A classic migraine is characterized by temporary narrowing, vasoconstriction, of the blood vessels in the head. Some persons experience a warning of the impending migraine. They see streaks or wavy lines of light (scotoma), experience intolerance to light (photophobia), and feel numbness, tingling, nausea, and sometimes mental confusion.

The second stage of a migraine is dilation of the blood vessels, causing a throbbing, excruciating headache that sometimes may actually be seen as a pulsation on the forehead. Medicines that contract these dilated arteries may abort the headache.

The third stage, the steady headache, is caused by *muscle contraction in the neck*. Obviously, because the neck muscles can constrict the blood vessel feeding the head, a tension headache could set the stage for migraine as well as follow it. Some researchers have observed that the only difference between a migraine and a tension headache is the degree of conflict in the victims' lives.

Migraine is not fully understood, although it is known that there is frequently a family history and that stress can set if off, just as stress can set off a tension headache. Migraine may also be caused by ingestion of chocolate, red wine or irregular hours.

The ideal answer, of course, in both migraine and tension headache is to cure whatever it is that is causing the psychological stress. You could help to identify the triggering stress by keeping a diary of each time you have a headache and what circumstances preceded it.

However, frequently the cause is subconscious. Or, even if you do know what causes the stress, you may not be able to avoid it because of the circumstances of your life.

There are a number of programs, which teach relaxation ranging from yoga to biofeedback. On your own, a warm bath, lying down in a quiet room, and just taking it easy may help.

Mild painkillers like aspirin are effective during a headache, and your physician may prescribe stronger medicines, such as tranquilizers or blood-vessel constrictors.

In any event, when something makes the hair on your head bristle, try to do some of the neck exercises in Chapter 13 to help you relax.

CHAPTER 9

SCALENUS ANTICUS SYNDROME

Another common neck problem which is often thought to be psychological but is actually organic is called the *scalenus anticus syndrome*, scalenus for the Greek word *skalenos* meaning "uneven" and *anticus* from the Latin "ante" meaning before, and *icus* meaning "more".

The scalenus anticus muscle is stretched between the third and sixth neck bone and the first rib. It crosses in front of the *subclavian artery*. The *subclavian artery* has branches which carry blood to the back of the brain, to the neck, the shoulders, and part of the chest.

The scalenus anticus muscle also crosses over the *brachial plexus*, a complex network consisting of nerves originating from the spinal cord, blood vessels connected to arteries from the heart and veins from the neck and arm. The brachial plexus is gathered together just behind the collarbone. It gives nourishment and movement to the chest, shoulders, and arms.

The scalenus anticus syndrome occurs when your scalenus anticus muscle squeezes the arteries and nerves underlying it, cutting off blood circulation and nerve sensation when you turn your head or raise your arm.

Take the case of the burly truck driver who was considered neurotic because of the puzzling nature of his symptoms. He said he had pain in both arms only when driving his truck, but did not have any discomfort when driving his own car.

The truck driver's symptoms were due to the fact that the truck he drove, had an unusually high, flat steering wheel which caused him to keep his arms elevated for prolonged periods. His car, on the other hand, allowed him to drive with his arms down.

A homemaker never experienced pain in her arm, despite a routinely strenuous round of daily activities, until she tried to paint the walls of a small room. She developed symptoms because she had to elevate her upper right arm for a long time while painting.

Schoolteachers, who write on blackboards, auto mechanics who work on raised cars, trap shooters, food servers in cafeterias, policemen, computer users, and many others suffer the scalenus anticus syndrome because of prolonged elevation of their arms during work.

Almost all victims of the syndrome complain of persistent pain extending from the neck into the upper extremity and fingers. The pain is often described as dull and aching, but it may also be sharp and burning. Frequently, routine household duties such as sweeping, dusting, and mowing the lawn may set off the attack. The suffering is also made worse by turning the head and weakness of the arm may occur.

Compressed Artery At The Base of The Neck

The *vertebral-basilar* artery syndrome, in which the artery at the base of the skull does not receive enough blood to feed the brain. Obstruction of the vertebral arteries can result in disturbances of balance, loss of vision, hearing impairment, dizziness, fainting, and paralysis. The most common causes are hardening of these arteries, degeneration of the neck bones, rotation of the head, trauma, and pinching of the nerves by the scalenus anticus muscle.

If the scalenus anticus syndrome is not treated, the arms may become weak or numb. Doctors usually recommend the correction of poor posture, weight reduction in obese patients, and proper support of pendulous breasts. Patients are sometimes benefited by sleeping on two or three pillows, and/or sleeping with a pillow beneath the shoulder.

Severe pain may be helped when a physician injects an anesthetic into the scalenus muscle in the neck.

Should all else fail, surgery may be necessary to cut the muscle and release the pressure on blood vessels and nerves. When such an operation successfully frees the vessels and nerves, the results may be dramatic. There can be relief of dizziness, blurred vision, pain and numbness of the neck, shoulder, and arm. Even difficulty with memory and concentration may be caused by the compression of arteries and nerves.

Next time you raise your hand and you develop symptoms, consider the scalenus anticus syndrome.

Chapter 10

DIAGNOSIS

As mentioned many times in this book, neck problems may be obvious and easy to diagnose, or they may be very subtle and difficult to determine.

Two of the most important tools in any diagnosis are:

1) Your medical history.
2) The physical examination performed by your physician.

Your doctor will want to know whether you are under tension. Are you happy with your mate and children? Do you have in-law trouble? Do you like your role in life? Are you nervous about something? You don't want to undergo potentially uncomfortable and expensive tests only to have it later discovered that the pain was not in your neck but in your heart.

Daily habits must be explored. Is there a long, tense drive to work? Does the work involve bending over a computer or desk or painting a ceiling? What kind of furniture do you have at home? Do you read or watch television in bed? Do you hold the telephone cradled on your shoulder?

Do you suffer from insomnia or feel tired and stiff when you awake in the morning? Tension often takes its toll on the neck during sleep. Furthermore, the pillows or the mattress may be the wrong support for your neck or you may sleep in the wrong position.

> What's your posture like?

> Do you have a history of gastrointestinal disease or migraine headaches? Both are often associated with tension.

> Do you have a hormonal problem? Thyroid malfunction or insufficient sex hormones may cause muscle pain and neck bone problems.

> What kind of sports do you like? Are you just a spectator, which can be damaging to the neck? Do you like tennis or golf? Do you not indulge in any form of exercise? Are you an over conscientious housekeeper?

> Have you had operations or injuries in the past? If you've suffered a whiplash, for instance, that is very important to the diagnosis.

> What are your current complaints?

   ♦ Have you been injured?

   ♦ Do you warm up before doing your exercise?

   ♦ Was the pain sudden or insidious?

   ♦ Where does it hurt?

   ♦ When does it hurt - when you move, turn your head, sleep?

   ♦ Is it a sharp pain or dull pain?

   ♦ Does it extend down the arm or into the shoulder?

   ♦ Is there numbness or weakness in the arms or hands?

Have you found anything that gives you relief?

Your physician will assess your sensation, strength, and reflexes in various parts of your body to help pinpoint which nerves or what parts of your spine are affected. The doctor will perform a number of tests to determine your reflexes and the source of pain and how you move about. He or she will rule out other illnesses.

There are basically four basic neck syndromes:

1) *Nonradicular neck pain.* It is manifested to the area from the back of your head to the tip of your shoulder. This is the most common of the neck syndromes and usually is the result of either muscle spasm or disk degeneration. The nerve root is not involved.

2) *Radiculopathy neck pain.* Usually involves pain or abnormal sensations in the arm and/or hand such as tingling or burning. The most common cause is compression of the nerve root by a bone spur, a ruptured disk, or trauma.

3) *Cervical spondylotic myelopathy.* An unusual consequence of aging that may occur when a narrowing of the spinal canal puts pressure on the cord causing symptoms of numbness, weakness in the arms and legs and in coordination. There may also be loss of bladder and bowel control.

4) *Instability.* Slippage of the spinal bones or disks may be the result of trauma such as an automobile accident, a fall, arthritis or a birth defect. Any of the symptoms associated with the other three syndromes may occur.

To identify the cause of your symptoms, your doctor may then order X-rays. Ordinary X-rays will show only bone problems, although soft tissue abnormalities can be diagnosed from certain clues. A normal X-ray would show a bone with normal mineral density, a proper shape, alignment, and joint. A narrowed space between the bones may indicate a disc problem. Spikes or misshapen bones may indicate osteoarthritis and, of course, a fracture of the bone will show up in the X-ray.

Diagnostic Tests

There are a number of other tests that can be performed to determine the source of your pain in the neck. They include:

CAT Scan (Computed Tomography).

This is a computerized x-ray of your neck. You lie on a table with your head inside the machine which takes X-rays from many angles.

MRI (Magnetic Resonance Imaging).

This does not involve x-rays but rather a powerful magnetic field to produce a detailed anatomical picture of your neck and the structures within. During the study, you will hardly notice anything is being done but you must lie perfectly still if good films are to be produced.

Digital Holography System.

This is a new system, just coming onto the market at this writing, that combines Cat Scans and MRIs. They create a hologram, a three dimensional picture, of the spine and skull, reportedly making diagnosis of complex skeletal problems easier and more accurate.

Myelogram.

Infrequently used today, this involves an x-ray with a special contrast that highlights the spinal cord and nerves. The contrast is usually injected into the spine with a needle and then the X-rays are taken.

EMG and NCS (Electromyogram and Nerve Conduction Studies).

These devices test how your nerves and muscles are actually working together. EMG is a test which records the patterns of electrical activity of the muscles on a graph exactly as the electrocardiogram measures the activity of the heart. Every muscle in the body has its own unique pattern. When an EMG needle is placed directly on the skin, it conducts electricity through the muscles. Patterns emitted by the muscles can then be shown on the graph and doctors can determine whether there is damage to the particular muscle being tested. The EMG, however, is not restricted to one muscle. It can be used for an entire set. A doctor can check the entire neck area by viewing a recording of the impulses on the graph. He can determine exactly which muscles are involved in the malfunctioning. Doctors, of course, like to use the EMG because there is no danger involved. Using the machine takes a great deal of skill and cooperation. It does not work unless there is absolute silence. Interference of an airplane flying overhead or a train passing by can negate the results of the test. A soundproof room is usually employed. There are some patients who are too tense and nervous to allow accurate testing with the EMG.

Experiments with the EMG have been, most fruitful in contributing to the understanding of neck pain. A German physiologist actually showed that repeated tensing of the muscle results in a definite loss of length. The muscle actually shrinks; and when you are suddenly required to stretch it, it cannot do the job and reacts by going into spasm or, even worse, by tearing.

Two English physicians studied tension pain with the EMG. They found when the muscle contracts, it produces a weak electric current; the intensity of the current is in proportion to the degree of muscle contraction. They attached electrodes to "painful" muscles and to "normal" muscles in the same person. They then put the subjects through interviews expressly designed to stir up tensions. As the interviews proceeded, they noticed that normal muscles started to tense but then relaxed quickly. The muscles that produced the pain, however, not only started to tense during the interview, but tensed even more afterward, bringing about pain at the peak of contractions.

In summary, you can see how important telling the doctor everything can be. If you accurately describe your pain and the circumstances that cause it, you may avoid unnecessary tests and expense. But if your doctor does recommend the tests, you should now understand why they are necessary.

CHAPTER 11

HOW TO GET RID OF A PAIN IN THE NECK

If you have a simple neck strain without too much discomfort, there are a number of things you can do for it on your own. *If however, the pain persists, becomes more severe or recurs, see your family physician!*

The objective of treatment is to:

➤ Relieve pain and muscle spasm.
➤ Reduce inflammation.
➤ Protect the injured part to allow healing.
➤ Rebuild muscle power and restore a normal range of motion and function.

Should you take to your bed?
This is controversial. Some physicians say that the patient should be kept moving at all costs since stiffness and atrophy are increased by lack of action. But bed rest during the acute phase allows you to relax and to prevent further damage to

the injured part while it heals. The head is heavy and lying down reduces compression and pain in the neck. Your periods in bed should not be prolonged, half an hour to an hour, because muscles quickly deteriorate if they are not in action.

Some Like It Hot

Perhaps the most useful treatment in neck pain is heat. Soak in a warm bath, stretching out with the back of the head supported by rolled towels or a cervical pillow, with the warm water as high as possible so it covers the neck. In between baths, or if baths are not possible because of pain and disability, towels soaked in warm water or special commercial collar packs can be applied to the neck every two hours.

Moist heat is the best, but an infrared lamp can relieve mild discomfort and enhance relaxation. Shortwave diathermy is sometimes used for relief of deep pain, particularly that due to osteoarthritis. A professional should perform this.

Some Like It Cold

To every rule there is an exception, and some patients do better with cold than with heat. After trauma and during the acute phase of neck pain, application of cold to the neck for five to ten minutes at a time may reduce pain and swelling. Cold applied to the skin can reduce muscle spasm and associated pain because it cuts down on local circulation and metabolic rate as well as the rate of electrical output of the nerves. It anesthetizes the skin. Cold may be applied by placing ice in plastic bags, fastening the bags, and then wrapping them in a thin towel. The packs should be applied for fifteen minutes every two hours or so. Massaging the neck muscles with ice is another effective method of using cold. It may produce faster results, but it may also be uncomfortable unless the ice is enclosed in a plastic bag so that it can't drip.

Going to cold extremes

Ethyl chloride, a refrigerant gas, can be sprayed on the skin to freeze it and anesthetize it. Muscle spasm is then relieved and the patient, under a physician's supervision, moves the anesthetized part, helping to reduce stiffness and congestion. Sometimes a single ten-minute treatment is all that is needed. In other cases, it has to be repeated several times.

Ultrasound

Ultrasonic waves have a frequency too high for us to hear. By vibrating at eight hundred thousand cycles per second, a layer of tissue two to six inches deep receives a mini-massage. These vibrations increase the blood supply, stimulate metabolism, and produce a painkilling effect. Usually they are given in a series of eight to twelve ten-minute treatments, forty-eight hours apart.

Injection of anesthetic

Cooperation between the patient and physician is used to locate the so-called trigger points of pain. As the physician palpates the skin of the neck and shoulder, the patient tells him when he has reached the exact point which, when pressed, sends pain shooting down the shoulder and arms. An anesthetic is then injected directly into the trigger point. The local anesthetic works by interrupting the pain reflex. It paralyzes the pain receivers and senders. It relaxes the muscle spasm and improves the blood supply to the area.

This technique can be used in the base of the skull to greatly relieve headaches caused by tense neck muscles. (See Chapter 8.)

Injection of the anesthetic also allows the patient to move without pain. Since nature thrives on movement, this is beneficial to the neck structures. The effects of the injection may last for days or for months. The injection may be repeated when necessary.

Massage

Massage can help relax stiff muscles, particularly after heat has been applied. The muscle should be grasped between the thumb and fingers with a kneading motion. You may also find relief with a battery or electrically operated massage device available at a pharmacy or specialty store. Massage improves blood flow and promotes a feeling of well being. Too vigorous a massage, however, may increase tenderness and pain, so it should be done gently.

Neck collars

It is better not to use a cervical collar for a prolonged period if it can be avoided because the immobilization only weakens the muscles, causing atrophy. It is important that the collar chosen be of the proper type and fit, since such devices come in many different varieties. Muscle atrophy can start within 24 hours after trauma or immobility.

The type of collar recommended depends upon the degree of immobilization desired, although no neck brace can completely immobilize the neck. If minimum movement is indicated to reduce mechanical stress on the joints and strained or torn ligament, and to allow the painful muscle in spasm to relax, then a stiff plastic or molded leather collar should be employed. The collar may or may not need a chin plate, but it should be lined with felt to prevent pressure discomfort. It is very important that it fit properly. The back of the collar should be placed right below the back of the skull and, to avoid pressure and discomfort, should not rest on the two small protuberances at the back of the skull.

The chin should not be elevated to cause the neck to be hyper-extended.

If it is necessary to give only minimal support and remind the patient not to overextend his neck too much, then a soft foam collar is recommended. Such collars also come in a variety of shapes and sizes and should be fitted properly to the patient.

The neck brace should be used continuously until all symptoms have subsided, and then it can be gradually discontinued.

Sometimes back braces as well as neck collars are recommended to improve posture.

The most important things to remember about artificial supports of the neck are that the support must be fitted properly and that it should be worn according to a physician's instructions, since prolonged use can cause damage and atrophy of the neck muscles.

Cervical traction

Traction may be applied periodically or continuously in either a sitting-up or Lying-down position. Constant traction for a fracture is usually done in a hospital, produces some immobilization of the neck and helps to relieve muscle spasm and pain. Correctly applied, it straightens the cervical spine and enlarges the openings of the nerves to relieve compression or irritation of the nerve roots.

Intermittent traction can be done at home and, in some instances, is even better than constant traction. It can be adjusted to the weight, period of traction, and period of relaxation desired. The traction and relaxation act as a sort of massage leading to reduced muscle spasm and more effective subsequent traction. Because it is only intermittent, greater weights can be used with intermittent traction. The amount of traction is controversial, but many recommend starting with fifteen to twenty pounds and gradually increasing to about thirty-five pounds several times a day until free of symptoms.

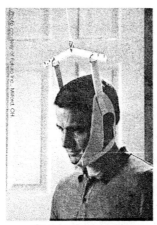

Traction sets for the home include weights, halter, pulley ropes, and a suspension unit. The weights are on a pulley and the traction unit can be placed over a door. The patient sits in a chair with a cloth strapping setup which fits under the chin. The weights exert pressure on the chinstrap pulling the head upward according to the weights on the pulley.

Cervical traction

Transcutaneous Nerve Stimulation (TNS)

Electrodes are applied locally to the neck in specific anatomical sites. Relief of pain and reduction of swelling can be achieved in about 30 minutes.

Medications

There are a number of pharmaceuticals that will help relieve pain in the neck. Nonsteroidal anti-inflammatory drugs (NSAIDS) are widely used. Aspirin belongs to this category as well as Advil® and Naprosyn®. They are often effective in reducing the acute inflammatory stage but should be used with care. Aspirin as well as the other NSAIDs may cause bleeding. Tylenol and other acetaminophen compounds are not anti-inflammatory but can relieve pain. Again, none should be taken to excess because they can also have side effects such as liver problems.

Oral and injected steroids may be effective in acute and severe inflammation and swelling. A class of compounds that includes certain drugs of hormonal origin, such as cortisone, can have serious side effects and should be used for only a short period.

Not everyone agrees that muscle relaxants are useful for neck pain. However, certain mild tranquilizers do provide relaxation from tension and, therefore, relaxation of muscles. When muscles are in spasm, it stands to reason that a muscle relaxant would be useful.

In some cases, sedatives, tranquilizers, and antidepressants may be prescribed. When tension is relaxed, so is muscle spasm. The use of the appropriate-mood drug depends upon the symptoms of the individual. Mild sedation during the daytime for patients with acute neck injuries is usually employed because such patients are often extremely nervous and apprehensive.

Biofeedback - Taking Control

Biofeedback is a technique designed to reduce tension by the measuring of biologic responses not normally felt or measured. When alerted by the signal to a change in pressure or body temperature, a person makes an effort to somehow produce more of the change. As a result, greater control over biologic responses is gained. This technique can be very effective when used with neck pain. It often can enable a patient to reduce spasm and pain and maintain function. There are no side effects.

Exercise

Exercise is helpful in both preventing and treating neck pain (see Chapter 13).

Get Rid of A Person or Thing Giving You a Pain In The Neck

Biofeedback is one technique to help you reduce tension. Sometimes you may literally need to get rid of whomever or whatever is giving you a pain in the neck. As pointed out throughout this book, your neck is very vulnerable to tension. Picture a cat's back arched when it is frightened or upset and you can understand how your neck reacts to certain frustrating situations.

You probably already know your own particular "pain in the neck." If you are not sure, keep a diary for a month and write down the circumstances surrounding your neck discomfort. Take action. If you need professional advice or a change in lifestyle, do it!

Remember This!

Because the head is being constantly moved by the neck muscles, the healing process may be prolonged. Anxiety and tension only lengthen the healing time, so be patient.

CHAPTER 12

IF YOU NEED SURGERY

In some instances, it becomes necessary to operate to relieve pain and to restore the neck to normal function. An operation may be urgent if there is progressive weakness in the arms or hands. There are several operations that are performed, depending upon whether it is a herniated disc, bone spur with pressure on the spinal cord or a lesion. Factors your physician and you will consider include:

> ➤ The diagnosis
> ➤ Your age
> ➤ The length of time you have had the problem
> ➤ Your physical health
> ➤ Disability such as progressive weakness.

Removal of the Disc From the Front (Anterior Cervical Discectomy)

The surgery is performed to relieve pressure on one or more of the nerve roots or from the spinal cord itself. The procedure is done through the front of the neck. The removal of the offending disc is accomplished under general anesthesia.

In some cases, the space between the bones is refilled with

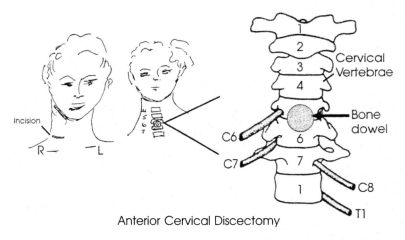

Anterior Cervical Discectomy

a small piece of bone that keeps the vertebrae apart and permits fusion of the bone.

Removal of Bone From the Front (Cervical Corpectomy)

As in the case of discectomy, the procedure is performed from the front of the neck. The surgeon removes a part of the neck bone (vertebrae) to relieve pressure on the spinal cord. One or more of the bones may be removed including the adjoining discs. The incision is usually longer than for removal of the disc, and the space between the bones is filled using a piece of bone or a metal plate. Because more of the bone is removed, the recovery period is generally longer than for just the removal of a disc.

Removal of a Disc and Bone Through The Back of the Neck (Cervical Laminectomy and Discectomy)

This operation is performed through the middle of the back of the neck. Through this opening, the surgeon pulls aside the muscles to expose the arch of bone called the *lamina*. The surgeon may also remove the bone around the spinal cord - *a laminectomy*. If the surgeon removes the bone around the nerve opening, that procedure is called a *foraminotomy*. After the nerve is located, it is moved gently aside and an incision is made in the outside covering of the disc through which the disc is removed.

Recovery from this procedure is longer than the anterior cervical fusion and is rarely done today except in cases were there are multiple areas of pathology or marked, progressive spinal cord compression (stenosis).

CHAPTER 13

HOW TO PREVENT A PAIN IN YOUR NECK

Prevention is always better than the best of cures. There is much that you can do to ward off a pain in the neck.

First of all, look in the mirror, preferably a three-way mirror used in clothing stores. What's your posture like? Are you hunched over or round shouldered?

We have become a nation of television watchers and computer users. The increase of the later has brought a skyrocketing increase in repetitive stress injuries (RSI) of the neck, shoulders, arms and hands. The job-related results of RSI cost business billions of dollars in insurance and treatment costs. Employers are trying to redesign work stations to adjust to each employees physical limitations but most experts agree a lot of the problem has to do with a worker's posture.

Studies at Loma Linda University have shown that the most prevalent fitness problem among young people is poor posture. Girls seem to thrust their heads forward and round their shoulders, a result of too much television watching.

Boys, who take part in more active games and carry and lift more than girls, escape this deformity until they get older and become less active. But both sexes exhibit the stance of old age much sooner than ever before.

When our shoulders are rounded, there is an excessive forward-head posture. This causes an increased outward curve in the neck often leading to pressure on the nerves.

Drooping of the shoulders results in over-extension of the neck, pulling on the nerves. Stooping makes the head go backward unless the neck is consciously held in position.

Some short people try to increase their height by walking with their chin up. This is the wrong position. It causes the neck to curve forward more than is natural, narrowing the opening for the nerves and eventually putting pressure on them. If the opening is repeatedly traumatized by physical and emotional tension, the nerve roots and their coverings become inflamed and swollen. They occupy a greater portion of the already narrowed nerve opening in the bone. The nerve becomes swollen and painful.

Close your eyes and touch your neck muscles. Then shrug your shoulders and touch them again. Can you feel the tension? Under tension, the muscles become painful and tender as we have pointed out before. By doing the exercises in Chapter 13 you can relax tight muscles. The following are some other things you can do to prevent a pain in your neck:

> While standing or sitting keep your neck drawn back and your chin tucked in.

> Use a proper chair that will support your arms and shoulders and help prevent the forward thrust of the neck. Proper arms on the chair are comforting.

> Write on a lapboard rather than on a high desk, but never write when under tension because it will increase

the strain on the arm and neck muscles.

➤ Adjust your car seat or sit on a pillow to avoid stretching the neck up and forward to see over the steering wheel. An armrest or cushioned support next to your arm while driving is restful.

➤ Do not slump in the chair. Sit up straight.

➤ If you must work on a high shelf or wash a window higher than your head, stand on a stool. Avoid reaching or looking up for any length of time.

➤ Squat don't stoop. Squatting is actually good for your hips. It is also good for your neck.

➤ When lifting an object, step close to it with one foot on either side. Then, using knee, hip, and back joints, lower your upper body downward and grasp the object. If you lift in this manner, you will be less likely to strain your neck or back.

➤ Do not carry a heavy shoulder bag. It causes pain in the neck by pulling down on the muscles of the neck.

➤ Do not sit at a table with your elbows resting on the table and your chin resting on your hands. It stretches the neck.

➤ Use reading glasses rather than bifocals. The location of the reading lens at the bottom of the bifocals causes the wearer to arch his neck upward and his head backward, compressing the nerve roots in the spinal canal at the neck. This produces the typical arm and neck pain and headache.

➤ Do not read in poor light.

➤ Avoid twisting to reach a phone and do not cradle the phone between your shoulder and ear. That's a real neck-straining habit. Use a speakerphone or headset if possible.

➢ Do not crane your neck. Activities including shaving, brushing teeth, applying makeup, or reading unfolded newspapers require the type of neck position that causes irritation of the nerve roots. This position is also a problem for people in a number of occupations. For example, a short radiologist who has to read films on a high view box; a homemaker who must read labels on food stored in counter cabinets; a scientist at the microscope on a high table; a mechanic who works under the car; and a paper hanger.

➢ Watch your leisure activities. Reading in bed with the head bent forward, ironing, viewing television while lying in bed, reading in a chair with feet stretched out straight can cause a pain in the neck.

➢ Don't be a weekend athlete - the kind that sits around all week and then on the weekend decides to play tennis, basketball and 72 holes of golf. Weekend athletes do not necessarily need to be playing games to hurt themselves. Gardening, involving prolonged stooping and repetitive movements like raking leaves often trigger attacks of neck pain because of fatigue of untrained muscles. Furthermore, working couples tend to put off their thorough housecleaning until the weekend. Making beds, lifting vacuum cleaners, stooping, awkward reaching and scrubbing can all set off a pain in the neck.

Computer Crunches and Creaks

More and more of us are spending time at work and at home typing away at our computers. The result may be what has come to be called *Repetitive Strain Injury (RSI)* or when it is work-related, *Occupational Overuse Syndrome (OOS)*. It may also be called - *Cumulative Trauma Disorder (CTD)* or *Work Related Upper Limb Disorder*. No matter what it is called, sitting in front of the computer for long periods of time can definitely cause a pain in the neck.

What happens when you over use your neck muscles or keep them in one posture or a strained position too long? You restrict the flow of blood. Without sufficient blood and the oxygen it carries, lactic acid may build up causing pain. Once a muscle is affected, its neighbors tense up, perhaps to relieve the load. As the tension builds due to repetitive, strained movement or inaction, less blood gets through and the cycle continues. As a result, you may feel tingling or numbness in your neck, arms or fingers. Your injury may be acute or chronic.

The first step is to make sure your computer environment is ergonomically right for you. Ergonomics is a fancy word for making sure your work environment fits your body and is comfortable. The following are some suggestions from experts in the field:

> Your keyboard should not be off to one side but in front of you.

> Your monitor should be at eye level.

> Frequently used items should be within arms reach from your keyboarding position. A document holder should be at the same height and distance as the screen so that your eyes don't need to change focus frequently.

> If you have to take dictation or make a number of calls, a speakerphone or a headset should be used to avoid bending your neck. Do not cradle a telephone receiver between you head and shoulder.

> Your elbows should form a 90-degree angle when hanging at your sides from your shoulders. They should be relaxed in a lowered position. Your seat height should allow your knuckles, wrist, and top of your forearm to form a straight line and your feet should be flat on the

floor.

➢ A chair with an armrest should be used and the seat should be ample for frequent changes in position. It should have a backrest that gives you firm support.

➢ There are other simple measure you may take to prevent cricks and creaks in your neck due to the use of the computer or just the plain old typewriter.

➢ Take a break at least every 15 minutes or 20 minutes.

➢ Shrug your shoulders and do some of the other easy neck exercises in Chapter 14 during your break or when you feel tension or stiffness while you are working.

➢ Periodically practice a relaxation exercise - whether it is just letting your shoulders and arms go limp or reciting a mantra. Remember that there can be a lot of pains in the neck at your place of work and at home.

Sleep Right Not Tight

One of the major problems with the neck is how to sleep in a good position. If possible, do not lie on your stomach because that position will not allow you to achieve a natural range of head rotation. The best position is lying on your side, with your arms down. If you develop pain or numbness in your arms when awakening, you may be sleeping with your head on them. Pin your sleeves to the sides of your pajamas to break the habit. Incidentally, you can cause this problem in others. You can make your bedmate's arm numb by sleeping on it; it is called honeymoon *paralysis*.

Other hints about sleeping without hurting your neck:

➢ A small down-filled or a soft fiber-filled pillow rather than foam rubber are best for sleeping. The weight of the head should depress the pillow and leave a somewhat higher support for the neck. You can push the edges of a regular pillow out from under your shoulder to under the neck. The pillow must be pliable. Or you can buy a special neck pillow. In any event, the pillow should fill the space between the shoulder and ear lobes.

➢ Sleep on a firm mattress. The best are made out of horse-hair, hog's hair, or felt; and they come without springs.

➢ Wear loose-fitting pajamas.

➢ Lying down backward from a sitting position or sitting up suddenly from a lying-down position can strain the neck.

➢ When arising in the morning from the prone position, roll to the side first and then push upward with your hands and legs to protect the head. After several hours of sleep in which the connective tissue has jelled, it is wise to rise slowly.

A Few Things You Should Also Avoid

Sometimes just simple changes can make a pain in the neck go away. Here are some of them:

➢ Grinding or clenching the teeth is frequently the cause of neck pain. Headaches in the front and side of the head may result. Even migraine headaches have been associated with poor bites. Chew gum to relieve tension. If you want to see how that works, look at coaches during a tense game.

➢ A brassiere with narrow shoulder straps can cause a pain in the neck as well as in the shoulders and back.

➢ Collars that are too tight or too high can cause a stiff neck or a tension headache.

➢ Never sit in one position for more than an hour. Driving a car for more than 60 minutes should be avoided.

Pull over to the side or stop at a refreshment place for a pause and a stretch.

If you make an effort to follow the advice in this chapter, you can greatly reduce your chances of having a pain in the neck.

CHAPTER 14

NECK CONDITIONING EXERCISES

You can keep a good head on your shoulders by conditioning your neck muscles. The stronger they are, the better they can do their job of holding your head up, and the less likely they will be to be strained or ripped. Even whiplash damage and recovery time can be reduced if the muscles are in good condition. The lack of neck muscle training may make you more prone to injury, even if you develop your other muscles to their maximum. If, for example, the muscles of your shoulders and back are substantially more developed than those in your neck, you could be more prone to neck injury during sports. The shoulder and arm muscles can overpower the weaker neck muscles and make them more vulnerable to stress, especially if you have a thin neck.

Strengthening exercises can often eliminate neck problems within four to twelve weeks.

The following neck exercises are intended to help you maintain and strengthen your neck muscles. Before you attempt these exercises, consult your physician. He or she will tell you whether they are appropriate for your neck condition. Do not do any exercises when you are suffering acute neck pain or if the exercise causes pain!

The exercises should be performed daily, slowly and evenly on both sides of the body. There should be a sensation of tightness in the muscles. If there is pain, use less force and reduce the number of repetitions. If pain persists STOP EXERCISING AND NOTIFY YOUR PHYSICIAN OR TRAINER.

Start out with the first exercise and then add an exercise each day until you have included all of them.

EXERCISE 1 Head Tilt For Range of Motion (ROM)

Keeping the shoulders level, tilt your head to the left and try to touch your ear to your shoulder. Hold this position for 3 seconds. Take a deep breath and exhale slowly. Return to straight position and repeat five times. Then do the tilt to your right. Hold for 3 seconds. Take a deep breath and exhale slowly. Return to straight position and repeat five times.

EXERCISE 2 Shoulder Elevations (Shrugs)

Sit erect on a chair and slowly take a deep breath and elevate your shoulders (shrug). Try to touch your ears with your shoulders. Drop your shoulders slowly and exhale. Pause. Then repeat 10 times.

EXERCISE 3 Head Rotation

Rotate your head clockwise 5 times (down - left - back - right). Pause, then repeat in the counter clockwise direction. This relieves muscle tension and improves coordination.

EXERCISE 4 The Windmill

Rotate your left arm in front of you like a windmill slowly and smoothly in a clockwise direction. Do it 10 times. Then do the windmill in the opposite direction. This is good for easing neck and shoulder pain due to arthritis. It also maintains neck and shoulder muscles and reduces stiffness.

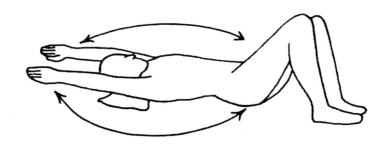

EXERCISE 5

Lie on your back on the floor with your knees drawn up. Place a rolled pillow, neck pillow, or rolled towel under your neck to support it. Take a deep breath and expand your chest to its limit. Then exhale slowly. Repeat this deep breathing exercise very slowly five times. Its purpose is to elevate the ribs and help you overcome the tendency for the upper back to press on the chest. It also strengthens the rib muscles.

EXERCISE 6

While in the same position as Exercise 5, turn your head slowly to the right, to the front, and then to the left. Repeat five times. This exercise limbers the neck muscles.

EXERCISE 7

In the same position as Exercises 5 and 6, making sure your feet are flat on the floor, press the small of your back hard against the floor. Tighten your buttocks and abdominal muscles. Breathing normally, tuck in your chin so that it flattens the back of your neck against the floor. Hold this position for a slow count of five. Then relax by releasing in order: your neck, shoulders, abdomen, and buttocks. The posture achieved by the spine in this exercise is the one you should aim for all the time. Chin in. Stomach in. Buttocks in.

EXERCISE 8

Still in the same position, lying on your back with your knees drawn up, slowly raise your arms six inches off the floor. Then slowly draw your arms over your head and touch your hands together. Then return your hands to your side. Repeat five times. If your shoulder muscles are painful, proceed very cautiously.

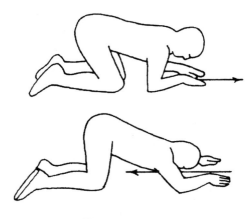

EXERCISE 9

Kneel. Place your hands and then your forearms on the floor, gradually pushing them along while you keep your head and back straight. This will stretch your chest muscles as you move away from your knees. Return to the kneeling position and then repeat the exercise three times.

Start out by doing one until you work up to five. Do not

proceed if you feel any sharp pain.

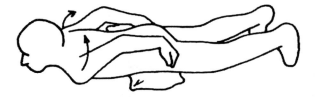

EXERCISE 10

Lie on your stomach with a pillow under your hips. Try to touch your shoulder blades together, then relax. This is a good muscle-relaxing exercise.

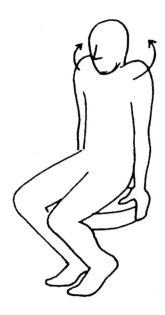

EXERCISE 11

Sit in a chair and try to touch your shoulder blades together as you look up at the ceiling. Return to normal position and pull your shoulder blades together as you look right and left. Repeat from the beginning. Look up at the ceiling as you pull your shoulder blades together: then right, and then left. All those who slave over a desk should do this exercise. It relaxes and stretches tense muscles.

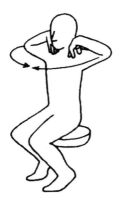

EXERCISE 12

While sitting in a chair, or standing, place your hands on your shoulders as in the old game of *Simon Says*. Touch your elbows, and then try to cross one elbow over the other. Repeat five times. This strengthens the shoulder and arm muscles.

Advanced Exercises

DO NOT ATTEMPT IF THERE IS ANY SORENESS IN THE NECK, SHOULDERS OR ARMS.

EXERCISE 13

Lie on your stomach. Rest your forehead on a folded Towel. Place your hands, fingers laced, behind your head. Slowly lift your shoulders and head off the floor. Then return to the starting position. If you feel any sharp pain, do not continue. Start out by doing this once and then gradually increase to five times. It will greatly strengthen the neck muscles.

EXERCISE 14

Lie on the floor on your back with knees bent and hands loose at your side. Raise your head and shoulders off the floor and bring them down slowly, and relax. This exercise strengthens the stomach, shoulder, and neck muscles.

Any Time, Any Place Exercises

EXERCISE 15

Sitting or standing, almost any place at all, turn your head to the left, then to the right, then rotate it in a circular movement several times a day.

EXERCISE 16

While sitting or standing, almost any place at all, draw your head back and tuck in your chin toward your chest several times a day, just as the Marines do in the old movies on TV. Take a deep breath and draw your shoulders back and up. Then lower them. Do this while sitting at a desk for a long time, while driving, while watching an event, or while riding in an airplane.

This last exercise relaxes your neck muscles and releases tension. If you can only do one exercise, do this one. As far as the neck is concerned, there is much to be said in favor of shrugging your shoulders several times a day.

GLOSSARY

Anterior - Front

Anti-Inflammatory - A medication for the reduction of the redness, heart and swelling that occur in infections and in other disorders such as arthritis. It is usually used as a painkiller.

Artery - Any one of a series of blood vessels that carry blood from the heart to various parts of the body.

Biofeedback - A technique designed to reduce tension by measuring the biologic responses not normally felt or measured. When alerted by the signal to a change in pressure or body temperature, a person makes an effort to somehow produce more of the change. As a result, greater control over biologic responses is gained.

Carotid Artery - There are two carotid arteries, one on either side of your neck to carry blood to your brain.

Cervical Spine - The seven vertebrae (bones) in the upper part of the neck.

CAT Scan - (CT) (Computerized tomography scan). A diagnostic imaging technique in which a computer reads x-rays to create a three-dimensional map of the soft tissue or bone.

Degeneration - Deterioration or worsening of a structure or condition.

Disc - The cartilage cushion found between the vertebrae of the spinal column. It may bulge beyond the vertebrae and compress nearby nerve roots, causing pain (slipped disc).

Fusion - The surgical joining of vertebrae with bone or metal.

Herniated Disc - Condition in which gelatinous disc material slips or bulges out of position and puts painful pressure on the surrounding nerves or spinal cord.

Joint of Luschka - Only recently have these vertebral joints been shown to be, instead, clefts in the fibrous tissue forming the circumference of the disks and not truly joints at all.

Laminectomy - Surgical removal of the rear part of a vertebrae in order to gain access to the spinal cord or nerve roots, to remove tumors, to treat injuries to the spine, or to relieve pressure on a nerve or the spinal cord.

MRI (magnetic resonance imaging) - Diagnostic test that produces three-dimensional images of the body structures using powerful magnets and computer technology. No radiation is involved.

Muscle Relaxant - A medication that relaxes tense muscles or muscles in spasm. Many tranquilizers have this effect.

Myelogram - An x-ray examination in which injected contrast outlines the spinal cord and associated nerve roots to illustrate spinal tumors and other conditions affecting the nerves and spinal cord.

Nerves - Fibers that conduct impulses (messages) from the brain and spinal cord to the muscles and glands or from sensory organs to the brain and spinal cord.

Spasm - An uncontrolled contraction of one or more muscles.

Spinal Cord - Bundle of nerve fibers enclosed in the vertebral column (spinal bones).

Spinal Stenosis - Narrowing of the vertebral column, resulting in pressure on the spinal cord or nerve roots arising from the spinal cord.

Steroid - A class of compounds used to treat inflammation that includes certain drugs of hormonal origin such as cortisone. Steroids, while very effective, can have serious side effects, all of which relate to the length and level of dosage. Adverse effects include susceptibility to infection, bone thinning, muscle weakness, diabetes, high blood pressure, bruising, increased pressure on the brain, psychotic reactions, hairiness, menstrual disturbance, cataracts and kidney disorders.

Stroke (Cerebral Vascular Accident) - Loss of muscle function, vision, sensation or speech resulting from brain cell damage caused by an insufficient supply of blood to part of the brain.

Transcutaneous Nerve Stimulation (TNS) - Electrodes are applied locally to the neck in specific anatomical sites. Relief of pain and reduction of swelling can be achieved in about 30 minutes.

Vagus Nerve - Literally "the wandering nerve" because it has such a wide distribution in the body, the vagus nerve connects the stomach to the brain and is involved in other autonomic functions such as breathing and heart rate.

Vertebrae - The 33 bones composing the backbone or spine.

Vertebral Artery - There are two vertebral arteries running up the back of your neck that carry blood to your brain.

About the Author

Arthur Winter, M.D., is a neurosurgeon and director of the New Jersey Neurological Institute. Ruth Winter, M.S., is a columnist and author of books on popular health and science. Their previous books include *Brain Workout, Eat Right, Be Bright* and *Build Your Brain Power.*

0-595-34920-X

Printed in the United States
38919LVS00002B

9 780595 349203